ARMY MEDICAL
OFFICER'S GUIDE

Army Medical Officer's Guide

Maj. Peter N. Fish,
MD, USA

STACKPOLE
BOOKS

"There are two groups of people in warefare—those organized to inflict and those organized to repair wounds—and there is little doubt that in all wars, and in this one in particular [World War I], the former have been better prepared for their jobs."

–Harvey Cushing, MD, 1916

Copyright ©2014 by Stackpole Books

Published by
STACKPOLE BOOKS
5067 Ritter Road
Mechanicsburg, PA 17055
www.stackpolebooks.com

This book is not an official publication of the Department of Defense or Department of the Army, nor does its publication in any way imply its endorsement by these agencies. The views presented are those of the author and do not necessarily represent the views of the Department of Defense or its Components.

Printed in the United States of America

10 9 8 7 6 5 4 3 2 1

First edition

Cover design by Tessa Sweigert

Library of Congress Cataloging-in-Publication Data

Fish, Peter, 1965–
  The Army medical officer's guide / Peter Fish, MD, Major, US Army
National Guard. — First edition.
      pages cm
  Includes bibliographical references.
  ISBN 978-0-8117-1184-5
1. United States. Army—Medical personnel—Handbooks, manuals, etc.
2. United States. Army—Officer's handbooks. 3. United States. Army.
Medical Corps. I. Title.
  UH223.F57 2014
  355.3'450973—dc23
                        2013035261

Contents

Preface

This book is modeled after the *Army Officer's Guide* (*AOG*), a must-read for newly commissioned Army officers for more than seventy-five years. While the *AOG* covers information that is absolutely essential to all Army officers in general, US Army medical officers are a unique breed and deserve an additional guide of their own.

This book explains the customs and regulations governing Army life, gives an overview of the structure of the Army's medical assets, discusses some of the heritage of the Army Medical Corps, describes the roles and responsibilities of an Army medical officer, and details the administrative, operational, and tactical aspects of the job. Much of the information included here has been gathered from active and retired medical officers who acquired their information through years of experience. Because much of this information is opinion—albeit well-informed opinion—offered by subject matter experts, it is not officially sanctioned by the US Army. In places where Army regulations and policies apply, the appropriate publications are listed. In addition, a list of relevant publications appears in Appendix D.

Every effort has been made to be complete and correct in this first edition of the *Army Medical Officer's Guide*, but readers may find errors and omissions. We invite you to contact us with corrections and submissions so that we can continue to improve this guide for future medical officers.

This book is intended for newly commissioned medical, dental, veterinarian, and allied health officers, all referred to as *medical officers* in this book. Military medical officers differ in several ways from the officers in the other corps. First, like the judge advocate generals (JAGs), who are military lawyers, they typically commission after obtaining their professional training. Although some physicians attend the Uniformed Services University of Health Sciences (USUHS), the military medical school, most medical officers receive their training as civilians. Some join while attending civilian medical, dental, or veterinary school, and some during residency, but most are directly commissioned after completion of a civilian residency. Second, most medical officers join the military at an older age than other Army officers.

Finally, they are commissioned at a rank higher than other Army officers without having any understanding of the basics of military life, which other officers have gained by moving up through the ranks. In short, Army medical officers are afforded privileges because of their unique skills but don't yet know of their unique responsibilities that warrant the special treatment.

Because new medical officers have not yet attended basic training and probably have had limited exposure to military life, they haven't learned the culture and rules of the Army. Thus they are entering a bewildering world of different language, clothes, laws, and priorities. To further complicate the transition, newly commissioned medical officers often innocently wear their uniforms incorrectly and make cultural gaffes without correction, as they outrank most of their patients and colleagues, and in Army culture it is considered impolite to correct people of higher rank. The rest of the Army tolerates these errors because of the value and scarcity of medical providers, often brushing them off with the comment "Oh, that's just the doc." Despite the leniency given to medical officers, these errors are still embarrassing to the individual and to the Medical Corps. You are not expected to behave and look like a career battle-hardened soldier, but you should look and behave in a way that is consistent with Army traditions, standards, and values. This book should help you with that.

Acknowledgments

One day in 2003, a man walked into the clinic on Stewart Reserve Air Force Base, wearing the rank of lieutenant colonel. As an accomplished endocrinologist, professor of internal medicine, and medical residency program director, this man had earned the rank that was pinned on his beret, and yet he bore the look of a new recruit. This man had recently been directly commissioned as a lieutenant colonel, and though he was essentially a raw recruit, no one had oriented him to the ways of the Army. After I helped that man—Colonel Richard Pinsker, MD—get his footing in the Army, he became my medical mentor, friend, and eventually colleague after he prodded me to attend medical school. Colonel Pinsker has been an inspiration to me on two tours, throughout medical school, and for this book.

This book could not have come to fruition without the support of my friends and colleagues in the 466th Area Support Medical Company, NY Army National Guard; the 102nd Infantry, CT Army National Guard; and the many enlisted soldiers, officers, civilian contractors, and patients who have educated me over the past fifteen years, both here and overseas.

I thank Colonel Timothy Connor (Ret.), my first commander, for whipping me into shape and teaching me the importance of basic soldiering skills for every single officer, regardless of rank and assignment.

I am forever indebted to Colonel Richard Green, DDS, commander of the 466th ASMC Combat Hospital. He had confidence in me when I had lost all of my own. His faith in me propelled me to succeed on that mission and on the greater mission of life.

My colleagues and friends Captain Jeff Avery, PA-C; Major Warren Sheprow, PA-C; Major Brian Rockwell; Lieutenant Colonel Peter Goetches, PA-C (Ret.); Colonel Glenda Shern, PA-C (Ret.); Colonel Craig Meinking, PA-C (Ret.); Lieutenant Colonel Edward Bonk, CRNA; SSG Jeff Lord; 1SG Jerry Loya (Ret.); Colonel Jamie Green, DDS; and Chuck Lappan, LTC (Ret.) alternately supported and taunted me through the past decade on several continents, in war and in peace. They are my family and deserve credit for the innumerable ways in which they have supported me and this project.

Colonel John Haynie (Ret.) shepherded hundreds of medical providers, including Colonel Pinsker and myself, through the rapid mobilization process for OEF and OIF deployments. His knowledge and motivation were invaluable to all of us.

SSG Erin Girdler, Indiana National Guard, is an inspiration in so many ways. An outstanding mother, soldier, and wonderful human being, her professionalism and attitude about life have motivated me more than she will ever know.

Thank you to Adam Foster Cohen at Military Credentialing Solutions for clarifying the important and complex process of establishing military medical credentials.

Finally, special thanks to Kyle Weaver, Brittany Stoner, and the staff at Stackpole Books for their patient editing and shepherding throughout the process of producing this book.

I

The Army Medical and Medical Specialist Corps

1

A Brief History of Military Medicine

Men have been binding battle wounds for nearly as long as they have been inflicting them. In one of the earliest accounts of battlefield medicine, Achilles is said to have bound the wounds of his friend Patroclus during the siege of Troy. Despite that promising early example, however, military medicine progressed little for another three thousand years. Although surgeons had some success in treating battle wounds, physicians probably killed more soldiers with lancets and potions than they cured. Until the introduction of vaccines and antibiotics, disease was the ultimate victor in every war.

The brief overview that follows is deliberately skewed toward the achievements of the US Army. Of course, significant achievements were made by military physicians around the world, including those in the US Navy and US Air Force, but physicians who served in the US Army made some truly extraordinary advances, although credit for these achievements is conspicuously absent from medical textbooks. The point of this chapter is not to rectify these oversights or lionize US Army doctors, but rather to establish that service in the Army Medical Corps is an honorable charge, and when you perform your duties, you will do so standing on the shoulders of giants.

It was up to a non-medical officer in 1775, General George Washington, ironically later a victim of physicians who ultimately killed him with their blood-letting treatments, to order smallpox vaccinations for all of his troops in one of the earliest examples of preventive military medicine. Perhaps under the influence of Dr. Benjamin Rush, General Washington also ordered the establishment of the first Army hospitals. Further, at a time when soldiers in Europe were typically fed only salted meats or insect-infested biscuits, Washington, in a move that foreshadowed the establishment of nutrition sciences, ordered that soldiers of the Continental Army were to be fed daily rations that included fresh fruits, vegetables, and beans; fresh meat; and fresh water. This forward-thinking attitude about preventive medicine in the Continental Army was, as with many things in the American colonies, probably a reaction to the centuries of warfare and disease in Europe. Regardless of the reasons, the precedents established by Washington and his physicians in the Continental Army have been continued to the present day.

Over the next century, the Army Medical Corps and the US Public Health Service made enormous strides. The Army Meteorological Service was founded simultaneously with the Army Medical Department (AMEDD) in 1818 to study the association between weather and disease, when Army physicians observed that malaria struck during the hot summers and influenza during the cold months. In 1833, Dr. William Beaumont, an Army surgeon who became known as the "father of gastric physiology," published *Experiments and Observations on the Gastric Juice and the Physiology of Digestion* after observing and experimenting for a decade with a patient with a fistulated gunshot wound. The Library of the Surgeon General's Office (now the National Library of Medicine, the largest medical library in the world) was established in 1836 to consolidate the most current medical research into one institution.

The carnage of the American Civil War (1861–65) again forced battlefield physicians to innovate. At that time cautery and amputation were the treatments for gunshot wounds, and, while effective, were very painful methods of treatment. What is not well known, however, is that surgeons in both Union and Confederate field hospitals used ether and chloroform anesthesia. Because blockades limited the supplies available to Confederate surgeons, they developed the first anesthetic mask, which used far less chloroform than a saturated rag placed over the nose, thus introducing anesthesia to tens of thousands of soldiers, journalists, and civilians who previously did not know of its existence.

A young surgeon's apprentice in the Union Army, Dr. Benjamin Howard, noted in a letter to the Army surgeon general that patients with gunshot wounds to the chest fared better when their sucking chest wounds were occluded. His recommendation is used to this day to prevent pneumothoray from penetrating chest wounds, and the procedure is taught to combat medics.

The American Civil War was heavily photographed, and the newly invented telegraph allowed for rapid press coverage. The widespread coverage of the battles led to public outcry about the casualties strewn across the battlefields, sometimes left there for days at a time. In response, President Abraham Lincoln appointed Dr. Jonathan Letterman, then the medical officer in charge of the Army of the Potomac, to devise a plan for evacuating wounded soldiers from the battlefield to hospitals. The system of trained and pre-positioned litter carriers, ambulances, train cars, and steamships that Dr. Letterman devised to evacuate patients from the battlefield was first tested in the aftermath of the Battle of Antietam, where ten thousand Union soldiers lay wounded. His patient evacuation system proved so successful that it became the basis for the modern-day Emergency Medical Services (EMS) and MEDEVAC.

Many other Army medical officers made their names during the Civil War. A surgeon in the Union Army, Dr. Gurdon Buck, operated on facial wounds inflicted in battles with the goal of improving not only function but also appearance. His achievements in reconstructing the faces of wounded soldiers earned him the title of "father of plastic surgery." Dr. Mary Walker, a civilian physician, volunteered to serve in the Union Army but was rejected because women were not permitted to serve in the Army (nor, indeed, were women accepted as physicians in most places at that time). Refusing to accept the rejection, she had a uniform made and reported for duty at a field hospital. She subsequently treated soldiers on both sides of the battle lines, was captured and put into a notoriously squalid Confederate prison camp, and returned to work on the front lines when she was released. She later was awarded the Medal of Honor for her service to the country. To this day, Dr. Walker remains the only woman to have received the Medal of Honor.

While not a physician, Union general Oliver Howard was a founder and the namesake of Howard University College of Medicine. Major Alexander Augusta, MD, was the first of approximately twelve African-American physicians to serve in the Union Army during the Civil War; was a professor of anatomy at Howard University College of Medicine; and was a staff member at the Freedmen's Hospital in Washington, DC, where he was the first black hospital administrator in US history.

Although Pasteur's germ theory had not yet been published, British nurse Florence Nightingale had introduced hygiene to field hospitals during the Crimean War (1853–56), which dramatically lowered the rate of wound infection and disease. Her well-publicized achievements and lobbying by Dorothea Dix and Clara Barton, two of the founders of American nursing, persuaded the US Congress to authorize the appointment of nurses in the United States Sanitary Commission and then the Army Medical Department in 1861. In 1901, the Army established the Nurse Corps as a permanent department, and by World War I, more than twenty thousand nurses were actively serving in the Army. Their service had a profound influence on the development of nursing, as many of these veterans went on to become teachers and faculty members of nursing colleges. The Yale School of Nursing was the first independent, university-based school of nursing in the United States, and its first dean, Annie Goodrich, was an Army Nurse Corps veteran.

The turn of the century was an extraordinarily productive time for the Army Medical Corps. Army Surgeon General George Sternberg published the first American textbook on bacteriology in 1892 after discovering the etiologies of malaria and lobar pneumonia. The first recipient of the Medal of Honor was an Army physician, Dr. Bernard Irwin, for valor in the face of the enemy in 1861 (though he did not receive the medal until 1898).

While field hygiene reduced some enteric diseases and wound infections, typhus, typhoid, yellow fever, and malaria remained huge adversaries, killing and incapacitating far more soldiers than enemy bullets. In 1900, Major Walter Reed was dispatched to Cuba with a team of physicians and researchers to determine whether yellow fever was caused by swamp gases or mosquitoes. When they discovered that mosquitoes were the cause, a massive campaign to eliminate mosquito breeding grounds was initiated, and the field of medical entomology was established. The man who ordered that research and the mosquito-eradication campaign that followed, Colonel Leonard Wood, MD, was a Harvard Medical School graduate who had joined the US Army in search of adventure and rose in the ranks to become the secretary of the Army. Colonel Wood was the first person to undergo surgical removal of a meningioma, with the procedure performed by a young Army surgeon named Harvey Cushing.

Around the same time that Walter Reed was doing his research, physicians at the Armed Forces Institute of Pathology were pioneering the use of X-ray machines in military medicine. Just three years after X-rays were discovered, Army physicians in 1898 developed a technique for using X-ray in the field to locate bullets embedded in patients.

In 1908, General Wood established the Medical Reserve Corps, which became the US Army Reserve in 1910. That same year, Major William Darnell, MD, developed a technique for chlorination of water, which effectively wiped out cholera in the armed forces.

The year 1917 saw the beginning of US involvement in World War I, and as with all wars, it led to further advances in medicine. Sadly, the first US casualties were a physician and a medic killed by an enemy artillery shell. Harvey Cushing, now known as the "father of neuro-surgery," volunteered for action as a battlefield surgeon in the Army Medical Corps during this period. The Army Specialist Corps was established in response to the onslaught of returning wounded veterans, in order to study and implement physical therapy. Nutritionists were added to the Medical Service Corps (MSC) to study and improve soldiers' rations. The new field of psychiatry was challenged by the legions of "shell-shocked" or "battle-fatigued" soldiers who had spent years in trenches living in mud and being bombarded by artillery. "Shell shock" and "battle fatigue" are now known as Post-Traumatic Stress Disorder. A shortage of soldiers on the front lines during WWI forced French physicians and psychiatrists to send "shell-shocked" soldiers back to the battle after only a few days of rest in the hospital. Their observations that rapidly redeployed soldiers actually fared better than those who were kept out of battle were a pivotal discovery. Rapid redeployment of soldiers who exhibit battle-related stress reactions is currently practiced with positive effects. Additional observations by field surgeons and shortages of supplies led to the development of low-volume trauma resuscitation. Traction splints for femur fractures were developed when army surgeons observed that these injuries had an 80 percent mortality rate when left untreated.

Medical research by physicians and scientists continued on the home front as well. In 1918, Major Reuben Kahn developed the first blood test for syphilis. Observations about the effects of TNT on munitions workers in England and the United States led to the discovery of the cardiovascular effects of nitroglycerin.

After the war, observations of soldiers who had been exposed to mustard gas weapons led to the development of methotrexate for cancer treatment. Facial plastic surgery was again advanced because of the numbers of severely disfigured soldiers in need of corrective procedures languishing in veterans homes. Observations that the physiological effects of flying at high speeds and altitudes caused US Army pilots to suffer from illnesses and sometimes experience crashes led to the establishment of the field of aviation medicine.

Dentists had made their first appearance on the battlefields during the Civil War, although only on the Confederate side. The Union Army did not contract dentists until the Spanish American War in 1898. The first full-time dentist was appointed in the Army in 1901, and the Dental Corps was permanently established in 1911. By World War I, dentists were being commissioned as first lieutenants and an Army dental school had been established. During that war, Army dentists treated more than 1.3 million patients in England, France, Belgium, Germany, Russia, and Poland.

An Army dentist played a heroic role in World War II. Dr. Benjamin Solomon, DDS, began his Army life as an enlisted infantryman, left the service to attend dental school, and then signed up again when World War II began. While serving in the Pacific on the island of Saipan, Solomon was called to the front lines to replace the battalion surgeon, who had been killed by the Japanese. As he was treating patients in the role of a field surgeon, the Japanese overran his treatment tent. Solomon single-handedly fought off the wave of attacking Japanese soldiers while his medics and patients escaped. He was found the next day slumped dead over a machine gun with a pile of more than eighty dead enemy soldiers in front of him. Dr. Benjamin Solomon was posthumously awarded the Medal of Honor for his act of valor in protecting his patients and fellow soldiers.

World War II produced so many medical advances and heroes that they can only be mentioned briefly. Some of the items mentioned were developed by civilian physicians and researchers but demanded by the war effort and implemented by the US Army. Among the notable advances were the first use of dehydrated blood plasma for trauma resuscitation, the first widespread use of penicillin and sulfa drugs, and the first use of aeromedical evacuation. Dr. Charles Drew created a blood banking system in response to the demand for whole blood in Army and Navy field hospitals. Other developments included PABA sunscreen to prevent sunburn in shipwrecked sailors, and mepacrine and chloroquine for the prevention and treatment of malaria (quinine was unavailable because the Japanese controlled all the islands on which the quinine-producing cinchona tree grew). DDT insecticide was developed to eradicate mosquitoes and fleas among soldiers and civilians; typhus was rampant in soldiers and civilians in postwar Europe, and malaria produced more casualties than enemy action in the early days of World War II in the Pacific. Widespread use of tetanus vaccinations in all soldiers and sailors virtually eradicated tetanus, which had ravaged the wounded soldiers who had fought in the manure-fertilized agricultural fields of France and Germany.

The Korean War followed just a few years later, and the medical lessons learned in World War II were applied in those battles. The Mobile Army Surgical Hospital (M*A*S*H) was first fielded in Korea, as were the first helicopters dedicated to evacuating casualties directly from the front lines to these hospitals. The Huey helicopter, which was the backbone of Army aviation in Vietnam and is still in use today by the US Marines, was originally developed as a medical evacuation aircraft. The addition of helicopters to the patient evacuation system still based on Dr. Letterman's 1860s plan increased the survival rate for soldiers who made the trip from the front lines to the hospital from 75 to 98 percent.

While medical technology was not greatly advanced during this war, Army medics (as well as Air Force medics and Navy corpsmen) were trained to perform or assist in lifesaving surgical procedures to further increase soldiers' survival. Thus, medics learned to apply anti-shock trousers and to perform venous cut-downs, needle thoracostomy, cricothyroidotomy, and escharotomy. The Army medics and Navy corpsmen who returned from World War II and Korea were so skilled that they were recruited into the first physician assistant (PA) programs, established to address physician shortages occurring in the United States in the late 1950s and early 1960s. In 1965, Duke University launched the first PA program, followed quickly by the University of Washington, Alderson-Broadus College, and Yale University School of

Medicine. Army PAs were initially warrant officers but became commissioned officers in 1992. PAs now serve in the Army Medical Specialist Corps, and having proven their value and skills for more than forty years, they perform medical and administrative missions at all levels in the Army with virtual autonomy.

The wars in Iraq and Afghanistan saw the introduction of new medical technology and techniques, increasing the rates of survival from what previously had been lethal wounds. Every soldier is issued hemostatic agents, tourniquets, and antibiotics, allowing individuals to treat themselves or their companions and to self-administer medications immediately after being wounded. Improved communications have increased evacuation speeds, and wounded soldiers arrive in combat hospitals for lifesaving surgeries, often within the hour. On the homefront, rehabilitation and prosthetic development have advanced to such an extent that soldiers with what once were incapacitating wounds are returning to duty with prostheses.

Only 1 percent of the American population have served in the Iraq and Afghanistan Wars, but the remaining 99 percent are benefiting medically from the sacrifices of the wounded and the medical providers treating them and from the lessons learned from them. Every time you put on the uniform of an Army medical officer, be mindful of these sacrifices and your duty to honor and treat those who served.

For more information on the history of medicine in the US Army, visit *history.amedd.army.mil*.

PATHWAYS INTO THE ARMY

The Army is always in need of medical providers and has set up multiple ways for them to join the service, providing generous financial incentives to do so. Aspiring candidates have such a large number of options, in fact, that explaining them often results in a glazed look of confusion. To make matters worse, candidates usually approach regular Army recruiters, who don't know anything about the Medical Corps and frequently don't even know to refer these candidates to specially trained medical recruiters.

The three biggest misconceptions held by both candidates and regular recruiters have to do with age, physical fitness, and medical conditions. Indeed, for regular soldiers who seek enlistment, there are strict criteria in these three categories, but none of them apply as strictly to medical providers. Medical providers can join the Army at any stage of their civilian careers, as the age limits placed on other military officer candidates do not apply to them. Candidates in their forties and fifties are often concerned that they will not be able to handle the physical demands of an Army position. In fact, the level of conditioning required of officers is linked to their age and is entirely manageable. Exceptions

Pathways into the Army

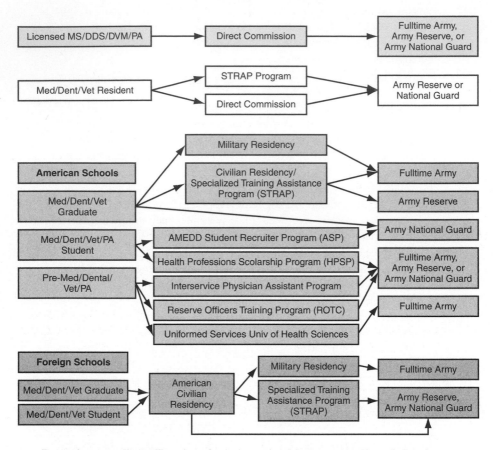

Becoming a medical officer in today's Army is a bit more complicated than it was in the past. This chart depicts the different pathways available to candidates pursuing officer's commission in the AMEDD.

to the rules can be made and waivers written for some medical conditions, such as hypertension, asthma, and certain orthopedic procedures, as long as they are controlled. The only requirement that is absolute is that candidates for the Officer Corps must be US citizens.

If you have picked up this book, you are already well on your way to deciding whether you want to be an Army medical officer. Thumb through the rest of this volume, and if it feels right to you, locate and speak with a medical recruiter. For information on the Active Army or Army Reserve, visit *www.goarmy.com/locate-a-recruiter.html*, and for the Army National Guard, see *www.nationalguard.com/careers/medical-professional-officer*.

2

Heritage, Customs, and Courtesies of the Army Medical Corps

No historical records or references have been found of customs and courtesies specific to the Army Medical Corps. This is unfortunate, as the Medical Corps has been in existence since the days of the Continental Army, and it would seem that there must have been traditions among the medical providers deployed to battlefields across the world over the centuries since. Unless they are somehow resurrected, perhaps from letters and memoirs, they will remain unknown. This chapter focuses on those customs and courtesies of Army officers that extend across all the branches.

As a medical officer, you will get considerable slack from personnel in the other branches with regard to uniform and behavior. Few officers are going to correct a medical officer who is out of line, because when medical services are required, the medical officer is often the only one who can deliver. In this setting, it is easy to become complacent in your behavior and abusive of the rules. You may, however, run into sergeants major who don't cut slack for anyone and will correct your appearance and behavior. Don't fight with them; they are right. Medical officers must set a high standard not out of fear of correction, but because it is the right thing to do. Although you can get away with a lot as a medical officer, you should not take advantage of this. Make the effort to learn the culture, courtesies, and uniforms. Your efforts will be noticed, and you will gain tremendous respect from your colleagues in other branches.

This does not mean that you have to lose your humanity and individual personality, but it does mean that you should be aware that people are watching you and that your behavior can have negative ripple effects on those over whom you have authority. It is on this basis that certain behaviors are expected of you and some are prohibited.

OFFICER BEHAVIOR

When you wear the rank of a commissioned officer, your behavior is held to a higher standard. Those in certain professions, such as health-care providers, police officers, and judges, are given privileges in exchange for the greater responsibilities they bear, but they are also highly visible and therefore expected to behave with decorum. Your superior officers expect you to perform to a high standard, your fellow officers expect you to adhere to the same high standards as they must, and junior officers and enlisted look to you to set an example. Your behavior and appearance in front of the troops influence the way they behave and set the climate of your medical facility.

COURTESY

Courtesy is essential in the military. Pick up a copy of the *Army Officer's Guide* to learn the basics. In addition to learning whom to salute and from whom you should expect salutes, there are rules of behavior that every soldier is expected to follow and that separate the professionals from the amateurs.

How to Correctly Perform a Hand Salute

Before the instance arrives to render the salute, stand or walk erectly with head up, chin in, and stomach muscles pulled in. Look squarely at the person to be saluted. If you are returning the salute of a soldier, execute the movements of the salute in the cadence of marching, *one*, *two*. If you are saluting a superior officer, execute the first movement and hold the position until the salute is acknowledged, and then complete your salute by dropping the hand smartly to your side. The junior soldier executes the first hand salute, holds the position until it is returned by the senior, and then executes the second movement.

When saluting, be sure to have the thumb and fingers extended—a protruding thumb is especially objectionable. Keep your wrist bent (the hand and wrist should be in the same plane) and hold your upper arm horizontally.

Saluting

Saluting is the most fundamental of courtesies in the Army. Officers and enlisted below you are required to salute you when they are within three

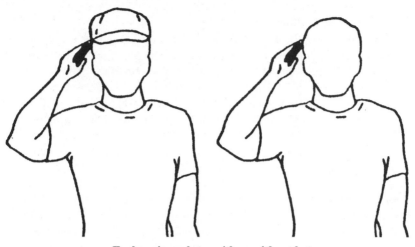

Exchanging salutes with or without hat

to five paces of you, and they are to address you verbally as well, with either a greeting or a unit motto, such as "Hellfighters, sir!" You are expected to respond with a salute along with an appropriate verbal greeting. The person initiating the salute is not permitted to drop his or her salute until you drop yours. Saluting is expected between services as well, and it is good manners between officers of allied countries. Soldiers who are smoking or talking on their cell phones are expected to stop, stand at attention, and salute. You will encounter young servicemembers who fail to salute you either because they are not paying attention or because they are testing you. They should be corrected on the spot.

Practice your salute, and deliver it briskly and appropriately to superior officers and in response to subordinates. A sloppy or missed salute is inexcusable and rude. When you are in uniform, you are expected to keep your right hand free so that you can salute without fumbling or hesitation. In other words, carry your briefcase or coffee in your left hand if you anticipate encountering other soldiers.

There are some exceptions where you are not required to salute, such as in the field or a "no-salute zone." You also are not required to salute when you are seated in a vehicle, such as when you drive through a military checkpoint and a guard salutes you, but it is polite to do so. When soldiers are in groups, only the most senior is required to salute. If civilians salute you when they see you in uniform, you are not expected or required to salute them in response, although you may do so if you choose. However, a verbal "Thank you" is generally a good idea, as their intent is usually friendly and honorable.

Standing at Attention

When a superior officer enters a room, stand and call junior officers to attention. Non-Commissioned Officers (NCOs) or sergeants will usually do this before you get a chance, but be alert regardless. You are not required to stand for NCOs, but if a sergeant major (SGM) or command sergeant major (CSM) enters the room, stand anyway; to have attained that rank, they have been in the Army for a long time and have earned their stripes the hard way by coming up through the ranks. SGMs and CSMs will have the ear of your superior, so show them respect even though they call you sir.

Verbal Greetings

You must address any officer of higher rank by his or her rank and name, and you should expect to be addressed that way by those of lower ranks. You may also address higher-ranking officers as ma'am or sir. Do not address them by their first names unless they invite you to do so. If they invite you to address them in some way other than their rank, it is expected that the informal means of address is to be used only when subordinate officers or soldiers are not around. When addressing subordinate officers around their subordinates, use their proper ranks and names so as to preserve their authority with their troops. If a senior officer addresses you by your first name, accept it and do not correct him or her. It may be a sign that the officer approves of you, but it could also mean the opposite. Either way, pay attention if you hear your first name uttered by a superior.

When addressing an officer of a different branch of the military, you are expected to state his or her rank correctly as a sign of respect. All branches except the Navy have the same ranks, so this is really only complicated if addressing a Naval officer. If there are no junior Naval officers around who can discreetly help you get their boss's rank right, address the officer as sir or ma'am until you can quietly and humbly admit your ignorance and ask him or her. Salute the officers of other branches and be prepared to return their salutes. Make sure your soldiers do the same.

Soldiers' names and ranks are right on their chests, but make an effort to learn their first names. The bonds you make with your troops by knowing their first names, as well as any personal information you can gather about their families and interests, are the seeds of friendship and help inspire their loyalty to you.

TREATMENT OF VIPS AND OTHER OFFICERS
General Officers

As an officer in the medical corps, you will encounter many other officers on a regular basis and will get to be on a first-name basis with many of them. Because they are your colleagues, you may become so comfortable with them that you grow complacent about your salutes and greetings. However, generals of every rank (general officers) must be saluted. In fact, even general officers' cars, if clearly identifiable with markings, must be saluted because they may be occupied. Most generals will immediately tell you to stand at ease, but failure to come to attention and salute is highly disrespectful. If you are treating a patient when a general enters your area, it is understood that you are to continue with your care. The general is likely to be more interested in the welfare of the soldier anyway, but you must still be respectful and address the officer as "General," "Sir," or "Ma'am."

Medal of Honor Recipients
In the unlikely but fortunate event that you meet a Medal of Honor recipient, you must salute them and call them sir or ma'am regardless of rank. These individuals have received the highest military honor in the land, and though they are unfailingly humble, they are to be honored. Even generals salute them. They are given priority on aircraft, at all military events, and for all services. It is your honor to give up a seat for them.

No one *wins* the Medal of Honor; servicemembers *receive* the Medal of Honor and are referred to as Medal of Honor *recipients*. This is an important distinction: they did not win a competition, but performed acts of valor to save the lives of their fellow soldiers at risk to their own—and often at the cost of their own—while asking nothing in return. To call them winners would imply that their comrades-in-arms were losers, which is disrespectful.

The Medal of Honor is approved by Congress and awarded by the president, but it is not called the Congressional Medal of Honor, as one frequently hears. There are four Medals of Honor, as each branch has its own. The award is properly called simply the Medal of Honor or is preceded by the name of the branch, as in the Army Medal of Honor.

Retired Officers
It is good form to refer to retired officers by their rank, salute them, and treat them with deference as if they are still active members. Retired veterans have earned that respect.

Addressing Other Medical Officers
You should address other medical officers by their rank and name until they invite you to do otherwise, or until you become friendly with them. Most soldiers call any combat medic or PA simply Doc, rather than Doctor. If this offends you, get over it. It has been that way forever and is entrenched in Army culture. Correcting these soldiers won't change

their behavior, and attempts to do so will make you look like a prig. Soldiers will address you by your rank, so you will almost never be called Doctor. Colleagues may address you as Doctor, but more often than not they will use your first name or rank. When in front of the enlisted, however, it is highly improper to use first names.

RELATIONSHIPS
Special Relationships
Special relationships are a constant source of problems for otherwise excellent officers. These include both romantic or sexual and critical or ostracizing relationships. If you have specific feelings toward a soldier and allow those feelings to affect your behavior such that you give the soldier special positive or negative treatment that is in contrast to how you treat other soldiers, you are in the wrong. Adultery is a crime in the Uniform Code of Military Justice (UCMJ), and it can lead to court-martial, demotion, and jail time. Fraternizing with soldiers of lower rank is considered behavior unbecoming of an officer and can also be prosecuted, even if both participants were willing. It becomes even more damaging if the lower-rank participant says that he or she felt compelled to participate because of your higher rank, in which case you face far more serious charges. There is a saying among soldiers that have been deployed that "what happens on deployment stays on deployment." Don't count on it. Emails, texts, tweets, and Facebook pages are all scrutinized by many eyes, and people get caught, no matter how slick they think they are. Think about it—if the head of the CIA can get caught, as in the situation involving a former Army general, you can too.

Command Relationships
If you are assigned to a combat arms unit, you as a medical officer hold a special position with the commander. At staff meetings, you or your medical superior sit at the head of the table to the left of the commander. Because you need to interview and examine patients, you have a private office, which may be a tent or trailer. You or your boss will usually be the highest-ranking member of the unit, sometimes outranking the commander. You know and share with the commander the personal issues of all the soldiers and officers in the unit; you are also isolated from the unit's chain of command, answering only to the commander. You are often the only person in a position to be the commander's confidant. If you consider the amount of responsibility the commander bears and the stress under which he or she operates, your role becomes even more daunting, since you are responsible for the physical and mental health of the person who is responsible for the lives of everyone

under his or her command. The commander must know that regardless of your personal opinions, religious beliefs, or political leanings, you are loyal to him or her and to the mission, and that he or she can rely on your confidence, discretion, and wisdom.

BEHAVIOR WHILE IN UNIFORM
Rules and Etiquette for Walking in Uniform
You are not permitted to eat, drink, or talk on a cell phone while walking in uniform. If you wish to engage in one of these activities, you are to stop in place while you do so. Wearing earbuds or earphones while in uniform is forbidden. Men are never permitted to carry umbrellas while in uniform, though they may hold an umbrella over someone else. Woman in uniform are permitted to carry an umbrella and a purse on a strap over the left shoulder.

When wearing a backpack, both straps must be on the shoulders. If carrying a bag with a shoulder strap, it must be on the left shoulder so as not to interfere with the salute. Further, the bag must be carried on the same side as the strap (i.e. the strap may not cross the chest).

When you are walking with an officer who is senior to you, it is proper to stand to the senior's left and one step behind, thus placing that individual in what is considered the place of honor. If you are traveling with a group, it is good form to travel in a loosely organized formation rather than as a disorganized pack.

Political Events
It is a violation of Department of Defense (DoD) and Army Regulations to wear a military uniform to a political event or to make public political statements while in uniform. Members of the US Army take an oath to protect the Constitution of the United States and thus take on the duty of protecting the free speech of all Americans without regard to their political persuasion. To wear a uniform while making a political statement is to imply that your opinion is that of the military service. You do not speak for the Army, and thus your statement would be fraudulent.

Hats, or Covers
Cover is the Army word for a hat. All Army personnel remove their covers when inside a building; the only exception is for soldiers who are carrying loaded weapons on guard duty. If you interact with Navy or Marine officers, you will notice that they wear their hats indoors when on duty. Follow the Army rules when you are in an Army uniform. When you are wearing a civilian hat out of uniform, it is still considered proper form to remove the hat when the American flag is raised or lowered, during the National Anthem, or at a funeral when Taps is played.

OFFICER BEHAVIOR DOS AND DON'TS

Do

Wear the appropriate uniform

Address soldiers by proper rank when on duty

Make sure the enlisted are recognized for their work
with awards

Salute appropriately

Praise in public, correct in private

Know your chain of command

Salute officers of other services

Learn proper ways to address officers (of all branches)

Listen to and learn from senior NCOs (much like new
doctors learn from nurses)

Don'ts

Don't eat, sleep, or take care of personal needs before
the enlisted

Don't correct officers or NCOs in front of their soldiers

Don't argue with an officer or senior NCO in front of
troops

Don't pull rank if you are clearly in violation of a
regulation

Don't overindulge in drink while in uniform

Don't cross in front of formations; instead, go around
back

Don't make racist or sexual comments in public

Don't have special relationships with the enlisted or
junior officers

Don't eat, sleep, or take care of any of your personal
needs before making sure that the enlisted are settled

Don't give orders to senior NCOs without an
explanation

Don't micromanage or smother senior NCOs or junior
officers

Don't undermine your missions or orders by being
cynical or negative

Don't complain or brag about accommodations; the
enlisted have it worse than you do

Don't jump chain of command

Don't correct junior medical providers in front of
patients; if they are doing something unsafe, stop
them and take them aside

Don't walk while talking on a cell phone or wearing
headphones or earbuds

FORMATIONS

For most military units, the workday and all missions begin and end with a formation. A formation is an organized group of soldiers standing at attention or at rest in rows ("ranks") and columns forming a rectangle facing the ranking NCO or officer in that unit. The soldiers stand in order of rank. Officers stand in a row behind the formation, also in order of rank, from the highest at the right to the lowest at the left. The purpose of this exercise is to allow the officers and NCOs to account for all the troops, inspect them, and make announcements. When you are standing in formation, it is bad form to talk, text, or do anything that distracts from the announcements going on at the front of the formation. If you arrive late to a formation, either discreetly enter the formation from behind or wait until it is over. Never cross in front of a formation; you should walk around behind it.

REVEILLE AND RETREAT

On military bases, the official day begins with the basewide broadcast of a bugle playing Reveille and ends with the bugle playing Retreat, which is Taps followed by the National Anthem. The flag is raised during Reveille and lowered during Retreat. If you are outside when you hear either Reveille or Taps, you must stop where you are and come to attention facing the flag, or the general direction of the flag if you cannot see it. When the National Anthem is played, you must salute if in uniform or remove your hat and place your hand over your heart if in civilian clothes or physical training gear. If you are driving on a base during Reveille or Retreat, you must stop your vehicle, turn off your radio, and sit at attention until it is concluded. If you are in a building, you may continue your duties uninterrupted.

MILITARY SOCIAL EVENTS
Promotion Parties, or "Wet Downs"

When an Army officer is promoted, it is traditional for a party to be thrown for the officer at a bar or club after the formal promotion ceremony. It is also traditional for that officer to pay for the drinks at that party and for fellow officers to brag about how much they are going to drink to "soak" the promoted officer. Keep in mind when attending or organizing a wet down that a recently promoted first lieutenant is not as well paid as a recently promoted colonel, so when you make him or her pay for your drinks, you might be taking money from his or her family. It is fine to tease the young officer, but use your judgment and pay for your own drinks as appropriate.

The tradition is borrowed from the sea services—the Navy, Marines, Coast Guard, and Merchant Marine. They call it the "wetting down" ceremony, and in addition to drinking and making toasts to their new officers, they throw them into the sea or throw seawater on them. The water portion of the ceremony helps the new officers approach their new job with humility as they enter a new rank. Tradition has it that dowsing the new sleeve stripe and rank device with water weathers it so that it doesn't appear so new. After all, who wants to be led by a brand new officer? Although the Army does not generally incorporate the water portion of the ceremony, it is at the discretion of the participants and is not prohibited. If you do intend to actually wet down the guest of honor, make sure that any cell phones and wallets are removed prior to the event.

Retirement Parties

Retirement parties in the military can be dining in/dining out affairs or they can be less formal. For servicemembers who have served more than twenty years, they tend to be formal affairs with presentations of awards, flags, retirement promotions, letters from dignitaries (or from the president, for service of thirty years or more), speeches, and gifts. Being invited to a retirement party is an honor. It is good form to research the retiring officer's career and to learn his or her spouse's name so you can congratulate them in person or offer a toast.

Weddings

Military weddings have become more popular in recent years, presumably because more servicemembers have been deployed. Though many take place at military chapels, this is not a requirement. In fact, the only features that define a military wedding are the presence of uniforms in the wedding party and the Arch of Sabers at the conclusion. As a guest at a military wedding, you are generally expected to wear your dress uniform, though you may opt for civilian clothes if you prefer. If you are a member of the wedding party, you will be directed accordingly.

The highlight of a military wedding is the Arch of Sabers. This tradition involves six to ten servicemembers in uniform. These servicemembers usually act as ushers during the wedding; at the conclusion of the ceremony, they exit the church before the bride and groom, collect their sabers (preferably matching US Army sabers), and assemble into two facing rows at the exit to the church. On the commands "Draw sabers, present sabers, arch sabers," members of the arch party draw their sabers with points up, place the hilts to their chins, and then extend their arms with the sabers crossing, edges up, above head level, forming an arch through which the bride and groom can walk or run. Before the couple can exit the arch, however, the two Arch Party members farthest from the door drop their sabers to waist level to stop the bride and groom, and then smack them on the behinds and say, "Welcome to the Army, Captain and Mrs. Jones!"

Funerals

Servicemembers killed in the line of duty, honorably discharged, or retired are entitled to military funerals. Depending on the circumstances and their rank at death, they may be entitled to honors, such as an honor guard, uniformed pallbearers, military chaplain, a twenty-one-gun salute, and the presence of a unit of soldiers. All military funerals conclude with the playing of Taps on a bugle and the presentation of a folded American flag to the surviving spouse or family members by a uniformed representative of the US Army.

As a guest at a military funeral, you should wear your Class A Uniform out of respect to the deceased and survivors and to show that the Army family is present. If the funeral is for a member of your unit, you should sit with other members of the unit. You have the option of wearing a black arm brassard on your left arm while traveling to, attending, and traveling from the funeral. (The relevant official publication is AR 670-1, Section 28-29.)

Members of the funeral party do not salute or return salutes while performing their duties. When they pass bearing the casket, you should salute the casket. When the casket is being lowered into the ground and Taps is being played, you should also salute. While the flag is being presented to the survivors, stand at attention.

If you choose to attend the wake in uniform, remember that you represent the Army and behave accordingly. The combination of grief, alcohol, and military uniforms can be explosive. If you observe behavior in another uniformed servicemember that does not reflect well on the military, because of either grief or alcohol or both, it is your responsibility to intervene and escort him or her away to cool off. Don't be the person who needs to be escorted.

Parades

Participation in parades is generally voluntary, although a commander may require it. The commander determines the uniform.

Formal Ceremonies

If you are invited to a military ceremony, the uniform of the day will be explained in the invitation. If you are asked to participate in an event involving a general, member of the US Congress, or someone from the

White House, you may be required to wear a particular uniform, along with specific accoutrements, and perform specific roles. You can find the details in DA Pamphlet 600-60, A Guide to Protocol and Etiquette for Official Entertainment.

Celebrations and Performances

Active, active reserve, honorably discharged, and retired servicemembers are permitted to wear their uniforms to social events such as celebrations and performances. When worn with a black tie, the Class A Dress Blue Uniform or Dress Mess Blue is considered to be equivalent to a tuxedo, and the Dress Mess White Uniform is appropriate for a white tie event. The Tropical White Uniform is also authorized until July 2014 for wear in hot climates or during the summer to social events.

Dining-In/Dining-Out

Formal dinners to celebrate victories and honor heroes are as old as warfare. The Roman legions, the Vikings, and the Knights of King Arthur's Court certainly engaged in victory feasting. Monasteries and universities also incorporated the tradition, building special dining halls for the purpose, through the military's banquets are more formal. For centuries, the British military has conducted regimental dinners during which soldiers and officers don their most formal uniforms and gather for highly ritualized and traditional feasts. The British officers fighting the Americans during the Revolutionary War brought their regimental dinner tradition with them, and it so impressed General George Washington that he began conducting them for the Continental Army. General Washington's initiative has been carried through to this day as the Army dining-in.

USAREC Pamphlet 600-15, Dining in and Dining Out Handbook, defines the dining-in as "a traditional formal dinner for members of a military organization or unit. It provides an opportunity for members to meet socially at a formal military function to recognize individual and/or unit achievements or any events that are effective in building and maintaining unit esprit de corps. In addition to offering good food and beverages, it provides an atmosphere in which unit tradition, history, and accomplishments serve as a base for building and maintaining professional camaraderie. A dining-in may be held to honor one or more distinguished visitors or to say farewell to departing members and welcome new ones. A dining-in should be viewed as an opportunity to enjoy the companionship of one's fellow soldiers rather than as a mandatory function. . . . Many still follow the old, lively pattern of dining-ins held by units during World War II. These usually include a period of fun and games after the formal program of awards and speeches." A dining-in is also an occasion for a military unit to celebrate its history, teach etiquette to younger soldiers and officers, and invite spouses and guests to share in the pageantry. If spouses, guests, or civilians are present, the event is known as a dining-out.

These banquets have had a recent resurgence in popularity, perhaps because Operation Enduring Freedom and Operation Iraqi Freedom veterans have an increased interest in military heritage. Regardless of the reasons, dinings-in are opportunities to put on Army dress uniforms and celebrate Army heritage. Each of the services, and each branch within each service, has its own specific traditions, but the basics of the dining-in are similar.

The dining-in/dining-out is an opportunity for the different branches to express unit pride through variations to their uniforms that are not otherwise authorized. Cavalry units wear Stetson hats, cowboy boots, and spurs with their dress blues; Airborne units tuck their pants into polished black jump boots; Artillery units replace the gold stripes on their pants with red ones; Engineers wear special "Essayons!" gold buttons emblazoned with the castle of the Army Corps of Engineers; and Irish or Scottish Infantry units wear kilts with their blue jackets. Soldiers may also elect to wear dress swords, capes (yes, they are authorized), full-size medals, drill instructor hats, and various other appurtenances. Retired soldiers are encouraged to attend in their uniforms, as are guests from other services and other countries' militaries. Nonmilitary guests should be advised that the dining-in or dining-out is a formal or black tie affair and they should dress accordingly.

The banquet is a formal multicourse seated meal served by professional waitstaff, often held in the dining hall or a rented banquet hall. The guests are expected to wear their best uniforms, along with their medals and ribbons, and to enjoy themselves while behaving in a formal and appropriate manner (think wedding reception). The meal is a ceremony that follows a specific program and is directed by the president of the mess, seated at the head table (usually the commander of the unit hosting the banquet), and the vice president of the mess, called Mr. or Miss or Ms. Vice.

The room is arranged with a head table facing an array of individual tables or arranged in a T with a long banquet table. Seated at the head table are the president of the mess, guests of honor, speaker, and chaplain. Spouses may be seated with the officiants if the banquet is a dining-out. The vice president is seated alone at a table facing the president so that they may openly dialogue and direct the sequence of events for the evening.

Organizers may elect to prepare a "missing soldier" table or place setting that is set apart from the other tables or settings. This is done to commemorate soldiers who were killed in battle, are missing, or are unable to attend because of injuries. No one sits at this table. During the toasts, the table is recognized and a toast is offered to the dead and missing.

It is common to provide each guest with a printed program of the evening's activities, which includes a list of mess rules. Over the course of the meal, guests, known as members of the mess, may stand, address the president of the mess, and in a good-natured manner, point out violations of the mess rules by other members of the mess—commonly such things as uniform infractions, discussing work, or bragging about medals—hoping to bring down punishments on their fellow soldiers. Punishments can include reciting poems, performing push-ups, drinking the grog, or small fines, which go to charity.

Depending on the occasion for the event, the number of guests, and the preference of the organizers, the event may be highly formal and conservative or it may be more boisterous. Similarly, it may include alcohol or may be dry, although alcohol is the essential element in the grog bowl ceremony, which is traditional and central to the event.

> **The Usual Sequence of Events at a Dining-in/ Dining-out:**
> Social hour/receiving line
> Call to mess
> Entrance of the official party
> Post colors/National Anthem
> Invocation
> Welcome and toasts
> Dinner
> Speech by the Guest of Honor
> Grog bowl ceremony
> Benediction
> Army song/retiring of the colors

A common feature of the banquet is an ongoing dialogue during the event between the president and vice president of the mess, directing the proceedings and discussing the various infractions committed by members of the mess and the penalties levied.

At the appropriate time, guests may rise and offer toasts to members of the mess. The initial toasts are formal and honor the country, the

Army, the command, and VIPs. Subsequent toasts may be serious and formal, but they can also be in the form of limericks or poems that poke good-natured fun at other guests.

The grog bowl ceremony is frequently a highlight of the banquet. At the appointed time, members of the mess gather around the bowl, and read aloud a narrative of the unit's history. At designated points in the narrative, alcoholic beverages that are symbolic of particular battles or achievements are added to the bowl. For example, participation in World War I might be signified by adding Bordeaux wine, and the Pacific Theater of World War II with sake.

For more information on the dining-in and dining-out, see USAREC Pamphlet 600-15, Dining-In and Dining-Out Handbook.

OTHER CUSTOMS
"Hooah"
"Hooah" (correctly pronounced "HOO-uh") is a word unique to the Army that soldiers use in many ways. It can mean "yes," "hooray," "toughness," or "ingenuity." Soldiers may use it as a greeting, a cheer, a personal quality, or an explanation, as in "Hooah, sir!" or "That humvee is not in good shape, sir, but with some extra oil and some hooah it might just get there." Counterparts in other services are the Marines' "Ooh-raah" and the British Army's "Huzzah!"

Coins
Commemorative coins have a long history in the civilian world, but they have become popular in the US military only in the past two decades. Senior officers and NCOs have the unwritten right to have special coins minted at their own expense that are unique to their organizations. Because coins are not regulated as awards and medals are, commanders and senior NCOs have the latitude to decide the circumstances under which they give away these coins. Typically, VIPs, commanders, or senior NCOs give the coins to enlisted soldiers as unofficial tokens of a job well done, although it is usually possible to purchase generic commemorative coins as well. When given as an award, the coin is slipped to the soldier in a handshake rather than presented publicly in a ceremony, thus adding a personal and secretive flair to the award.

Coins are often collected and traded. It is customary that if a servicemember sitting next to another servicemember in a bar puts one of these special coins on the bar, the other servicemember must respond by presenting his or her own coin as well or by buying a drink for the challenger. If the challenged has a coin, however, and presents it, the challenger must buy the drinks.

3

Missions, Purposes, and Organization

"To Conserve Our Fighting Strength": this five-word motto of the Army Medical Command sums up the fundamental difference between the goals of military medicine and those of civilian medicine. Ultimately, the goal of military medicine is to support the fight, wherever and whatever it may be. At the most basic level, providers in combat treat wounds and illnesses of combatants so that they can return to battle. Away from the battlefield, Army providers also treat and heal current family members who will never engage in battle, because the morale of the fighting forces and the continuity of the Army family demand that we do so.

Retired and disabled members of the Army are cared for by the Veterans Association Hospital System, which is a separate civilian organization but often confused with the Army medical system. President Abraham Lincoln made clear the moral imperative to care for these individuals in his second inaugural address in January 1865, when he talked about the task of rebuilding the country in the wake of the Civil War: "With malice towards none, with charity for all, with firmness in the right as God gives us to see the right, let us strive on to finish the work we are in, to bind up the nation's wounds, to care for him who shall have borne the battle and for his widow and his orphan, to do all which may achieve and cherish a just and lasting peace among ourselves and with all nations." The result was the establishment of national veterans cemeteries and the Veterans Administration.

THE ARMY MEDICAL DEPARTMENT (AMEDD) AND MEDICAL COMMAND (MEDCOM)

The Army Medical Command (MEDCOM) is responsible for the health of all current members of the full-time Army and Army Reserves and their families, and actively drilling Army National Guard. Depending on the current Medical Rules of Engagement, MEDCOM is also responsible for the care of civilians injured in battle as well. Thus, in addition to direct medical providers, MEDCOM also supports medical research, preventive medicine, medical technology research, medical education, and many other ancillary but critical disciplines. MEDCOM currently manages a budget of more than $13 billion and cares for more than 3.95 million beneficiaries—active-duty members of all services, retirees, and their family members. (For more information on MED-COM, visit *www.armymedicine.mil.*)

In general, MEDCOM is in charge of the organization and operation of Army medical facilities the world over, while the Army Medical Department (AMEDD) is in charge of the organization and training of medical personnel. MEDCOM also commands medical organizations that conduct medical research and are responsible for public health, medical materiel acquisition and distribution, and wounded warrior care. In short, as a medical officer, you work for AMEDD within MED-COM facilities using MEDCOM supplies and medical research.

The most senior position in the Army medical organization is the Army surgeon general. Each of the other military branches has its own surgeon general, as does the US Public Health Service. The Army surgeon general is the chief medical advisor to the secretary of the Army and commands both MEDCOM and AMEDD.

DIVISIONS OF MEDCOM AND AMEDD
MEDCOM is divided into five geographic regions—Europe, Southern, Northern, Western, and Pacific—and five additional nongeographic commands: AMEDD, Research and Materiel, Dental, Preventive, and Warrior Transition.

AMEDD is divided into eight subgroups: AMEDD Center and School, Medical Corps, Medical Specialist Corps, Medical Service Corps, Nurse Corps, Dental Corps, Veterinary Corps, and Enlisted Medical Career Management Fields. These subgroups are distributed between the full-time Regular Army and the Reserve Components of the Army, consisting of the Army Reserve, which is federally administered, and the Army National Guard, which is state administered. Currently, approximately 63 percent of all medical personnel in the overall Army are Reservists.

Army Reserve Medical Commands
In 1908, Congress formed the US Army Medical Reserve Corps, which in 1920 was expanded to become the US Army Reserves. The missions of the Army Reserves are operations, training, and support, which

effectively means that the Reserves do everything the full-time Army does, but with soldiers who train on a monthly basis. The US Army Reserves Command (USARC) is commanded by a lieutenant general at the Pentagon and currently has approximately 205,000 soldiers. Deployed medical forces from all components are usually under one of two Army Reserve medical commands: 3rd MEDCOM or 807th MED-COM.

Army National Guard Medical Personnel

Originating from the colonial militias beginning in 1638, the various state militias were standardized, reorganized, and renamed the US Army National Guard in 1903. The National Guard is under the control of state governors and available for activation by the governor in the event of state emergencies. In the meantime, the Guard trains to the standards set by the full-time Army, using the same uniforms, equipment, and training standards, and is subject to the same regulations. In times of national emergency, the president of the United States can activate the National Guard, at which time Guard soldiers become federal active-duty soldiers for the duration of the executive order.

The Air and Army National Guard units of each state have a state surgeon and a deputy commander for clinical services (DCCS), who command the state MEDCOM (not the same thing as Army MED-COM). The state surgeon and DCCS are direct advisors to the state adjutant general, who commands the Air and Army National Guards.

The Office of the State Surgeon has overall command of all medical personnel in the state, regardless of their specific location or assignment. On a day-to-day basis, medical officers follow the routine of their particular unit and answer to the commander of that unit. But while medical officers are under the immediate command of whatever facility they are assigned to, they are ultimately serving at the pleasure of the state surgeon and follow medical directives, guidelines, protocols, and assignments that come from that office.

Medical officers in the Army National Guard may be assigned directly to the state MEDCOM or to various medical and nonmedical units around the state. When assigned to the state MEDCOM, medical officers usually perform periodic physicals for drilling soldiers or staff Soldier Readiness Processing (SRP), during which soldiers undergo medical evaluations to prepare them for deployments (military missions) or redeployments (returning from missions).

Medical providers in both full-time and reserve components can also be assigned to positions in various tactical units, such as Infantry, Armor, Aviation, or Artillery. In these units, they serve as medical

advisors to the battalion or company commanders and are the supervisors for the combat medics. When assigned to these units, medical
officers go out into the field with the units when they train to practice
field medicine out of tents or the backs of vehicles, known as tailgate
medicine.

4

The Army Medical Officer

GENERAL DUTIES

When you take your oath as an Army medical officer, your responsibilities increase dramatically. As a civilian, your chief obligation is to your patient. As an Army officer, however, your medical decisions are no longer a private matter between you and your patient; your decisions now affect the mission of the soldiers you are treating, and by extension the US Army and the country. When you treat soldiers, you cannot assume that they can take time off from work and go home until they are better. Injured and ill soldiers have serious responsibilities that must be fulfilled on a strict timetable, either by them or by a replacement. If you send a soldier home, you may cripple that soldier's mission, which can in turn endanger a larger mission, potentially costing lives and endangering national security. It is your responsibility as a medical officer to learn that soldier's responsibilities, be in contact with his or her chain of command (CoC), and advise the CoC of that soldier's limitations and capabilities. In a sense, you must view a patient who is a soldier as a vital piece of equipment that must be repaired and put back into service as quickly as possible, and in the meantime used in some other way as much as possible.

Perhaps the most difficult concept for many physicians to comprehend is that the medical care of an individual soldier is not the top priority of an Army commander; the mission takes priority over everything else. Consider the simple fact that military commanders are authorized by the president and Congress to send soldiers to their death to accomplish missions. Put in that context, it becomes clear that operations will not stop even if they jeopardize the life of your patient. It is your job as a medical officer to advise a commander of medical situations, both individual and global, that may affect the mission. In addition, you are tasked with treating or evaluating sick and injured soldiers, performing physical exams, training your medics, and keeping your inventory and equipment up-to-date and functional.

31

MEDICAL INTELLIGENCE

You become a valuable asset to a commander when you offer medical recommendations that forward the mission while maintaining the health and fighting capabilities of his or her soldiers. In nonmilitary terms, you are the preventive medicine advisor to the commander, and your job is to research in advance the hazards presented by the conditions into which the soldiers will be inserted and how the risks can be managed. Those recommendations include control measures and observations about weather, insect and animal threats, food and water issues, hygiene, sleep and fatigue, medical resources and supplies, and plans for management of casualties. Your findings and recommendations are to be presented at planning meetings with the commander.

For example, it is useless to a commander to have a medical officer simply tell him or her that many soldiers will be hurt on a dangerous mission in the mountains. On the other hand, it is extremely useful for a commander to hear specifically from a medical officer, in the form of a Medical Threat Assessment Brief, that in preparation for the upcoming mountain mission, the medics are instructing soldiers on how to properly wear winter gear, and that based on the weather report and the upcoming winter storm, a 3 percent cold injury rate and a further 5 percent casualty rate from altitude sickness are anticipated. In preparation for the casualties, the medical officer would like to move an ambulance and aid station forward with the troops to rewarm hypothermic soldiers and return them to duty ASAP, because evacuation in the snow will be impossible. It is also useful for the commander to learn in advance that the medical officer will need a heated shelter, the troops will need high-calorie mountain rations and extra water, and cold-weather boots and sunglasses should be issued to reduce sunblindness and frostbite.

One of the most poorly managed risks in the battle space is fatigue. Since most physicians have trained in an environment of almost-constant fatigue, their perspective tends to be skewed as well, reasoning that if they could survive medical school while tired, soldiers can do their jobs tired as well. Multiple studies have shown, however, that more errors occur when personnel are fatigued. In the military, those errors include death from friendly fire, vehicle and aircraft crashes, and walking into ambushes. It is not helpful for a medical officer to advise a commander that his or her troops are tired. It is helpful, however, to advise a commander that the troops will be functioning at only 50 percent of their potential capabilities under the current work-rest cycle, and that the mission should be simplified to reduce mishaps. The Fatigue Avoidance Scheduling Tool (FAST), developed by the US Navy for aviators, allows a medical officer to plug a soldier's sleep schedules into a program that calculates his or her predicted performance capacity. It is available for free download to DoD personnel at *www.novasci.com/ index_files/page0003.htm*.

FIXED FACILITIES
Full-time or Regular Army medical providers are usually assigned to fixed facility hospitals and clinics. These hospitals and clinics are located on military bases and serve the entire military community. Members of the medical staff are augmented by civilians and Army Reservists who have been called up to backfill for providers who have been deployed overseas.

COMBAT MISSIONS
One of the appeals of military medicine is the variety of opportunities and adventures it affords. As an Army doctor, you will probably have the chance to travel to places you might otherwise not see and treat patients in environments you cannot imagine as a civilian. As a Regular Army medical officer, you are likely to be sent on an overseas mission at some point in your career. At today's high Operational Tempo (OPTEMPO), Reservists can expect a deployment as well. Medical officers are always in high demand and short supply, so if you specifically want such an assignment, there are plenty of missions for which you can volunteer. Full-time Army physicians and PAs can expect to be deployed on twelve- to fifteen-month missions at least once in their careers, their regular positions being backfilled by deployed Army Reserve providers. Army National Guard medical officers tend to get mobilized with their assigned combat arms units rather than being individually deployed as Professional Filler System (PROFIS) backfill, though they can volunteer for both overseas and stateside missions.

Combat deployment types depend on your medical specialty, your military training, and your rank. Surgeons will be deployed to fixed facilities with operating rooms, generally on well-protected and established bases, unless they are specifically trained for and assigned to a forward surgical team (FST). Full-time Army nonsurgical physicians, dentists, veterinarians, and PAs can also expect to be assigned to fixed facilities and placed in positions analogous to their practice in the continental United States (CONUS). Army National Guard medical officers are more likely to be assigned to forward bases in mobile medical facilities: an area support medical company (ASMC), forward support medical company (FSMC), or battalion aid station (BAS). When assigned to missions in combat zones, you draw extra pay, a significant portion of your income is tax-free, and you are eligible for combat medals and ribbons.

USERRA AND SCRA

If you are a deployed Reservist, you are also the beneficiary of rights and privileges of the Uniformed Services Employment and Reemployment Rights Act (USERRA) and the Servicemembers Civil Relief Act (SCRA; formerly the Soldiers' and Sailors' Civil Relief Act). Despite the flag waving that takes place when soldiers depart and return from war, they have often been victims of unscrupulous individuals in their absence. Even at the beginning of the recent wars in the Middle East, Reserve Component servicemembers returned home to find their jobs given away, their houses foreclosed on, and various other personal catastrophes. Laws have been on the books for many years to protect against some of these events, but the outrage that manifested from press reports led to a reexamination and bolstering of the old laws. USERRA and SCRA were the results of subsequent legislative efforts.

USERRA protects servicemembers' jobs in their absence, legally entitling them to any promotions and pay raises that were due to them while they were serving. Further, it is illegal for their employers to obligate them to use up sick time or vacation time to "pay" for their absence. An employer may hire a replacement for a temporarily vacated job but must open that position or an equivalent one to the servicemember upon his or her return. Employers are not obligated to pay the servicemembers in their absence, although some do as a patriotic act, recognizing that the extra duty performed for the country also incurs a pay cut for many individuals. (For more information on USERRA, see *www.esgr.mil.*)

SCRA protects deployed soldiers from various civil actions that could take place in their absence while deployed. Their property is protected from foreclosure or seizure until they return, and they are afforded special rights with regard to leases, mortgages, credit card loans, and civil suits. Upon presentation of deployment orders, deployed servicemembers must be released from leases on cars or apartments, interest on all loans must be reduced to 6 percent, and civil suits, including mortgage foreclosures, must be suspended until a specified period after the servicemember has returned from deployment. Unfortunately, there have been some high-profile examples of banks that foreclosed on houses of deployed soldiers despite the provisions of SCRA, but they have since been sued by the government and compensated the soldiers. (For more information on SCRA, see *www.justice. gov/crt/spec_topics/military/scra.php* or *www.dmdc.osd.mil/appj/scra.*)

It is important to understand that in order for SCRA and USERRA to be effective, the servicemember must notify employers, banks, creditors, plaintiffs, and courts by providing them with copies of his or her deployment orders prior to deploying. Once those orders have been

received, the servicemember is protected. Many banks now have departments dedicated specifically to deployed servicemembers and adherence to SCRA.

Employer Support of the Guard and Reserve (ESGR) is an organization formed to help Reserve Component servicemembers interact
with their employers to resolve conflicts or misunderstandings about
military service. ESGR representatives will visit employers to answer
questions and negotiate on servicemembers' behalf. ESGR also spon-
sors events to thank employers that have been particularly supportive.
The Bosslift (also BossLift) program, for example, enables servicemembers to nominate their employers as supporters of the Guard and
Reserve, whereupon the nominated individuals and organizations
receive framed certificates of appreciation and are invited to board a
military aircraft to observe an aerial refueling exercise or the like. For
details, see *www.esgr.mil.*

If a servicemember receives a notice that is not in compliance with
one of these laws or has difficulty with an employer, creditor, or court,
he or she should consult a judge advocate general (JAG, a military attorney) immediately. JAGs can be found on every major military installation for a personal interview. Further information is available at
www.jagcnet.army.mil/Legal.

DEPLOYMENT LENGTH LIMITS
Although they may volunteer for longer missions, National Guard and
Army Reserve physicians, dentists, and veterinarians may not be activated for longer than ninety days every two years, and PAs may not be
activated for longer than six months every two years. This law was
passed in order to protect doctors' practices, which can be badly dam-
aged by prolonged absences. Full-time Army medical officers can be
deployed indefinitely.

PEACE OPERATIONS AND NONCOMBAT SUPPORT
MISSIONS
Deployments can send you to areas where the United States and allies
are performing "missions other than war," such as Kosovo, the Horn of
Africa, Germany, or Cuba. You also may be called on for aid because of
natural disasters or for humanitarian assistance. These are noncombat
missions, so while you are performing an important role, you are far
less likely to treat combat injuries or be exposed to the dangers of combat. Natural disaster missions are often emotionally challenging, but
since your services are desperately needed, these missions are professionally and spiritually rewarding.

Humanitarian and Civil Assistance (HCA)

Army National Guard and Army Reserve medical units are sometimes deployed on missions that support civil authorities during natural disasters or for humanitarian assistance. Because the National Guard can be deployed by state governors, they are far more likely to be called up for blizzards, floods, hurricanes, or the like. If a natural disaster involves several states, federal property, or an act of terrorism, then the Army Reserves may also be called up to assist.

Simple humanitarian missions to underserved countries are often scheduled to align with the annual two-week training periods for National Guard or Reserve units so that medical personnel are able to bring their resources to medically underserved places in South America or Africa.

Medical Civic Action Programs (MEDCAPs)

In a Medical Civic Action Program (MEDCAP), doctors and specialists with equipment and supplies set up a temporary field clinic to provide limited medical treatment to the local population. MEDCAPs are generally narrow in scope and usually provide targeted assistance, such as inoculations, dental care, or eye exams. These can take place in CONUS, in friendly underserved areas, or even in hostile territory. MEDCAPs are "hearts and minds" operations.

SOLDIER READINESS PROCESSING (SRP)

Soldier Readiness Processing (SRP) is a program in which weekends are dedicated to readying soldiers for an upcoming deployment. Along with an administrative portion, the medical part of the process includes vaccinations, vision and hearing tests, a psych evaluation, and dental screening. Physicians and PAs also review medical histories with deploying soldiers, update their computer records, and address medical issues as they arise.

FIELD TRAINING EXERCISES (FTXS)

Field training exercises (FTXs) are just what they sound like: military training out in the open. Medical officers rarely get an opportunity to see soldiers practice their warfighting skills. Worse, medical officers rarely practice their own field skills, if indeed they ever learned them at all. Given the opportunity, all medical officers should go out to the field and get their hands dirty with a combat arms unit, help set up and run a battalion aid station, and sleep in a tent. It not only increases the confidence of the soldiers you serve in your loyalty and dependability, but also teaches you how they acquire their injuries.

HOME STATION TRAINING

Medical officers in the Reserves who are assigned to tactical units (medical companies or combat arms battalions) may not be tasked during drill weekends and are left to their own devices. You are expected to perform Officer Development Program (ODP) training on your own. This can consist of studying military or civilian medical material, non-medical military material, or training the medics and other medical personnel around you. Classes for the enlisted medical personnel are often repetitive, dull, PowerPoint lectures. Enlisted medical personnel are often grateful to have some hands-on training offered by a medical provider.

PHYSICAL EXAMS

If you are a full-time Army provider, physicals will be part of your daily routine unless you are a specialist. If you are a Reservist, the number of physicals you perform will depend on your regular duty assignment. Many Reserve medical officers spend every drill weekend doing only physical exams. If you are assigned to a combat arms unit, you will do periodic physicals for your soldiers who are going away to training schools.

For many healthcare providers, physical exams consume a significant portion of their time in the military. All newly inducted soldiers must receive a full physical exam prior to being accepted into the military. Unless you are assigned to a military induction center, you are unlikely to perform one of these physicals. Each soldier also receives periodic health screenings or checkups. Any soldiers going to a school that involves physical exertion must go through a physical exam that has requirements specific to that school. Soldiers that are injured, out of shape, or nearing retirement age require physical exams. Unfortunately, forensic exams are also not uncommon, so sexual assault exams and evidence collection procedures take place in military medical facilities, as well as exams for soldiers being court-martialed, entering prison, or having acute psychiatric issues.

AR 40-501, Standards of Medical Fitness, is the regulation that explains each of these exams, as well as the required paperwork. It is required reading for all medical officers and should be kept at hand for reference. Even if you are assigned to a position that does not require you to perform regular physical examinations, you must know the AR 40-501 regardless, because it defines the illnesses and injuries that result in Medical Board review, forced retirement, or discharge; details the paperwork to be filled out in the event of temporary or permanent injury; and describes the procedures for evaluating those medical conditions. Furthermore, officers will approach you with medical questions

about their soldiers or themselves, wanting to know how certain issues
will affect their duty or training. The answers lie in AR 40-501.

PULHES

PULHES is an acronym for general Physical condition (including dental), Upper extremities, Lower extremities, Hearing, Eyes, and pSychiatric condition. It is used to give a six-digit numerical evaluation score summarizing a soldier's fitness for duty under the Army's Physical Profile Serial System. Each category is assigned a number from 1 to 4, with 1 meaning fully capable and 4 meaning physically unable due to a medical or physical defect. Thus a soldier who is evaluated as 121121 is in excellent physical condition, may currently have a shoulder sprain but is expected to recover, has no other medical or psychiatric conditions, and wears glasses (2 in the eyes category). Every military occupational specialty (MOS) has a PULHES minimum requirement. The medical officer records each soldier's PULHES profile on DA Form 2808, Report of Physical Examination. Specifics about the PULHES system are explained in AR 600-60, Physical Profiling Evaluation System.

Discharge and Retirement Physicals

Expiration of term of service or estimated time of separation (ETS) refers to the date that an enlisted soldier is scheduled to be discharged from the Army unless he or she chooses to reenlist. Soldiers may retire from the military after twenty years of service and must retire if they reach age sixty-two. Before separation from the service, all soldiers must undergo a physical exam.

Command-Directed Physicals

Commanders have the ability to compel a soldier to undergo a physical exam. This may occur for several reasons: a commander may be concerned that a soldier has become injured but does not want to report it; there may be concern about an acute psychiatric event; or the commander may be about to initiate administrative or judicial actions against a soldier. You might observe that there is something wrong with a soldier and recommend to a commander that you or another provider conduct a medical evaluation. In this case, if the soldier denies permission for a medical exam, a command-directed exam may be necessary.

Chapter Physicals

Chapter physicals, also known as fitness-for-duty exams, evaluate physical issues that might make a soldier ineligible for retention in the military. "Chapter" refers to the specific chapters in the regulations that deal with medical reasons for discharging a soldier from the Army: AR 40-501, Standards of Medical Fitness, and AR 635-200, Enlistment Separations. These physicals may be requested when a commander observes that a soldier is seriously ill or injured, or in cases where a soldier is not performing his or her duty and the commander wants to rule out medical reasons for the shortcomings before beginning administrative actions. The soldier may have medical or psychological issues that the commander needs to take into consideration, and it is your job to determine whether any such issues exist and advise the commander.

Psychiatric Evaluations

If acute psychiatric issues appear to be preventing a soldier from performing his or her work, evaluation by a psychologist or psychiatrist is recommended as soon as possible after ruling out medical reasons for the behavior. If the soldier expresses a threat to self or others, an evaluation at the nearest emergency room is the best option, whether it is military or civilian. Commanders are not always sympathetic to psychiatric diagnoses, in which case the medical officer must be a strong advocate on the patient's behalf. A medical provider would do well to advise the commander that many stress reactions in military settings are short-lived and are successfully treated with a short respite and a return to the mission without stigma. When deployed, the combat stress teams are an extremely valuable and underutilized asset, and they are very focused on returning soldiers to assignments as soon as possible. In situations where the medical officer feels that a soldier needs someone to speak to, but no psychologist or combat stress team is available and the soldier's condition does not merit a MEDEVAC, the chaplain can step in and speak with the soldier as well. (For more information, see MEDCOM Regulation 40-38.)

School Physicals

While many schools and classes in the Army allow soldiers to attend if they have passed their Army Physical Fitness Test (APFT), the more physically and mentally demanding schools require special physicals for prospective students. Chapters 4 and 5 of AR 40-501, Standards of Medical Fitness, describe the requirements for each school. Chapter 4 deals exclusively with medical requirements for flying duty; these physicals must be conducted by a qualified Army flight surgeon or aeromedical physician assistant. Chapter 5 describes the physical standards for Ranger, Special Forces, Dive, Jump, SERE (Search, Evasion, Rescue), and Airborne Schools.

Forensic Physicals

It is an unfortunate fact that drug abuse, physical assault, and sexual assault take place among soldiers. In such cases, medical officers may need to perform forensic physicals.

Alcohol and Drug Abuse

Soldiers who are suspected of being under the influence of alcohol or illicit drugs may be brought to a military treatment facility (MTF) by officers or military police (MPs) for evaluation, but the urine or blood tests may not be released directly to the soldier's chain of command unless certain criteria are met. An officer must make a sworn statement that two people witnessed the soldier behaving in such a way as to raise suspicion of substance abuse, and the officer must make a statement that he or she is in the soldier's direct chain of command with a need to know in order to request a command-directed drug and alcohol test. This can be accomplished with a memo or sworn statement in the MTF. (Well-prepared MTFs have such a memo already written up, which the appropriate officer can fill in with specific details.) Any release of test results before receiving this statement is a violation of the soldier's privacy rights, and the evidence is inadmissible in an administrative hearing or court-martial. (See MEDCOM Regulation 40-51.)

Physical Nonsexual Assault

Physical assaults by soldiers on other soldiers are rare, and when they occur, soldiers are often reluctant to discuss them. The soldier does not have the right to prevent or delay an investigation by MPs or civilian police in this case, unlike with sexual assaults. Do not assume, however, that just because an assault was on a member of the same sex, sexual assault did not take place. It is important to ask the question explicitly, because the rules change completely if that has occurred. When performing an examination on a soldier who was nonsexually assaulted, take particular care to describe in the medical documentation the location, nature, and size of any injuries. Photographs are appropriate and very helpful. Make sure to put the soldier's name and date on every photograph and obtain a medical release before taking the photographs.

Sexual Assault

Sexual assault examinations are complicated procedures best handled by a senior medical provider. Large MTFs have a designated sexual assault clinical provider (SACP) on call to perform these examinations. A rape evidence collection kit is an essential tool in the procedure, as it contains the paper bags, labels, tarps, combs, lists, and other items necessary to collect the evidence. Proper examination requires privacy, proper lighting, and the assistance of a witness who is the same sex as the victim. The exam process can also be traumatizing for the victim, so the utmost discretion must be exercised. The sexual assault response coordinator (SARC), Victim Advocate (VA), or sexual assault clinical coordinator (SACC) for the base or area needs to be contacted immediately and should talk to the victim *before* the examination takes place. The victim has the right to waive or postpone an investigation by the MPs or police and may elect not to inform his or her Chain of Command, family, or colleagues. The military police and Criminal Investigation Department (CID) must be contacted to take possession of the forensic evidence, even if the victim has exercised the option not to pursue criminal investigation for six months. The SACC or SARC will notify the chain of command as necessary. It is strongly recommended that MEDCOM Regulation 40-36, Medical Facility Management of Sexual Assault, be on the required reading list of new medical officers.

TREATING OR EXAMINING ENEMY PRISONERS OF WAR
Enemy prisoners of war (EPWs) may be brought to an MTF for treatment of wounds sustained during capture or for an examination to document that they were healthy prior to bringing them for interrogation. Medical providers are obligated by ethics and regulations to treat EPWs in the same manner as they would American or Coalition soldiers. It is wise to have a witness and a guard present when performing the physical, as the prisoner may allege abuse during the examination or try to physically harm the medical staff. Photographic documentation of any physical findings for inclusion in the medical chart is advised, though care must be taken to avoid photographs of the whole face. All photographs not placed in the chart must be destroyed or erased.

PHYSICAL PROFILING
In the event that a soldier is disabled either temporarily or permanently, the medical provider must describe the occupational limitations recommended for the soldier on DA Form 3349, Physical Profile, or on the DA Form 689, Sick Call Slip, if the limitations apply for less than thirty days. Physical profiles can become complicated and have a serious effect on the mission. (Refer to Chapter 7 of AR 40-501 for details on how to properly execute a physical profile.) Generally, profiles can be temporary, lasting up to three months; long-term, lasting beyond ninety days; or permanent. PAs can write short-term profiles, but only physicians can write long-term profiles. Permanent profiles require the signatures of two physicians and a higher approving authority, such as a hospital commander or deputy commander of clinical services (DCCS).

MILITARY PATIENT CONFIDENTIALITY

Patient confidentiality is still the rule in Army medicine, but there are differences from civilian laws. First, military healthcare providers are subject to DoD 6025.18-R, the DoD Health Information Privacy Regulation (HIPR), which covers the same issues as the Health Insurance Portability and Accountability Act of 1996 (HIPAA). Both HIPR and HIPAA have a Military Exception Clause, which permits the medical provider to release soldier-patient information to that soldier's commander and chain of command if the information has a material effect on the mission to which the soldier is assigned.

MEDICAL CARE WHILE ON DUTY

Medical care for soldiers is dependent on the setting in which they are operating. Active-duty soldiers can present to any military medical facility if injured or ill, on duty or on leave, and receive treatment. In the event of an emergency, the soldier presents to the nearest hospital emergency department, even if it is civilian.

Reserve and National Guard soldiers who are injured or fall ill during their drill weekends are referred to local military or civilian hospitals rather than treated by medical officers because of concerns on the part of the Army about the medical liability of treatment by drilling medical providers. As the majority of medical issues that occur during a training weekend are minor, however, medical providers generally come to an understanding with their commanders about how to handle these issues to benefit the soldier while not cutting into training time. Deciding to treat certain soldiers on the spot rather than send them to a local hospital is a situation where officers may make decisions that may be against regulations or policies but are in the best interest of the mission. The military officers do so at their own risk, but it is their obligation as officers to weigh the risks and benefits to themselves and to the Army.

MEDICAL RULES OF ELIGIBILITY (MEDROE)

RoE are regulations that specify how service members are to interact with people or equipment outside the service (be they friendly or enemy), and who is eligible to be treated. The medical RoE define whom we may treat and how. The RoE may conflict with medical ethics, and may even conflict with the tactical situation at hand. As an Army Officer, it your duty to evaluate what to do in these situations and keep your commander informed and involved in the ultimate decision.

ROE also stands for Rules of Engagement, the battlefield regulations that define whom, and under what circumstances, a soldier may kill or capture. Each branch has its own RoE. For the Infantry Branch, the RoE define who or what can be engaged when and how with weapons.

The Medical Rules of Engagement are the regulations that define whom a medical provider can treat and how. MEDROE are set with military and political goals in mind and may not necessarily conform to the medical and ethical guidelines that you have learned. Regardless of whether you agree with them, they are the law and are enforced by the Uniform Code of Military Justice (UCMJ). If you have disagreements with them, discuss them with your tactical and medical commanders so that you all understand the issues at hand. There may be times when absolute adherence to the MEDROE is at odds with the commander's mission, in which case you may have to make some difficult decisions, taking into consideration mission priorities, the UCMJ, your personal biases, your oath as an officer, benefit to the individual soldier, and benefit to the unit.

For one example, at Camp Echo in Diwaniya, Iraq, the US Army MEDROE at one time prohibited the medical treatment of local Iraqis unless their injuries had been directly inflicted by American or Coalition operations. The local Iraqi hospitals had been looted and bombed, most of the Iraqi physicians had fled the country, and no medical supplies were available for those doctors who remained. In light of the local situation, the base commander decided to turn his head while the Army medical providers set up a clinic outside the gates and treated local Iraqi children. It was observed that during the months when the children were being provided with medical care, the base was not attacked with mortars. When outside Al Qaeda fighters violated that nonwritten agreement and attacked the base, causing the clinic to close, the next day the fighters' heads appeared on pikes outside the gate, apparently delivered by local Iraqis who had been taking their children to the clinic. Clinic care resumed. Later in 2006, however, when a new base commander arrived and vigorously enforced the MEDROE, forcing the clinic to close, mortaring resumed and did not stop for several months.

Although their actions had likely saved both Iraqi and Coalition lives, the medical providers could have been disciplined by their higher headquarters for violating the MEDROE at Diwaniya, because regardless of the circumstances, they had disregarded direct orders. It is unknown whether the chain of command did not know what was happening or chose to ignore it because they saw the beneficial effects. The history of war is filled with examples of situations where enforcement of regulations trumped reality. (See the case of the mutiny on the USS *Somers*, which partly inspired Herman Melville's novel *Billy Budd*.) The bottom line is that it is your obligation to follow regulations, but if you find that they don't seem to fit the local situation and are jeopardizing the mission, you should speak with the commander and consider the repercussions of acting otherwise.

In the case of Diwaniya, the medical providers and military commanders made decisions together about the MEDROE that had a direct impact on their missions. You cannot change the MEDROE. You must, as an Army officer, evaluate the MEDROE's impact on the local and overall mission, as well as on your patients, discuss any issues with your commander, and act accordingly.

YOUR PATIENTS

If you are assigned to an Army hospital, your duties as a medical officer will be very similar to what they would be as a civilian. You will be assigned to the department appropriate to your specialty, and you will see and treat patients. The main difference you may notice is that since your patients are either military personnel or their families, they will be remarkably punctual, respectful, and compliant. You will also have the luxury of treating patients according to their needs without having to worry about insurance concerns.

An important difference from civilian medicine, however, is that as a medical officer, you need to think like an occupational medicine doctor, since all of the soldiers you will see either were injured or became ill while on the job. Your goal is not merely to relieve their immediate pain or discomfort, but to get the soldier-patient functional and back to work as soon as possible with appropriate work accommodations. In other words, if you discharge a soldier from ambulatory care and simply write "Restrict to quarters," with no follow-up, you may severely cripple a mission. If you discharge your patients with specific work restrictions, abilities, and follow-up dates, most commanders will be able to adapt the workplace to allow these soldiers to continue to contribute their skills to the mission.

DA Form 689, Sick Call Slip, is used as two-way communication between a soldier's supervisor and the medical provider. On the left side of the form, the supervisor can tell you how the soldier was injured or became ill. On the right side, you write a note to the supervisor indicating the work status, restrictions, sedating medications, follow-up appointment, and any other pertinent information.

Even when you discharge soldiers from surgery, you need to consider the period of time during which they must be absolutely restricted from work versus returning to modified duty. Physical therapy (PT) and occupational therapy (OT) are available to soldier-patients without the restrictions imposed by civilian insurance companies, so you should consider PT and OT as means of speeding healing. In order to do that, you will need to know the specific physical and mental requirements of your patients' jobs, which could range from lab worker to mechanic to

Special Forces helicopter pilot. You will need to treat each soldier with his or her occupational demands in mind and in compliance with any medical treatment restrictions or guidelines that may exist.

The simplest way to learn the physical requirements and demands of your patients' jobs is to ask them. Alternately, you can look up their job descriptions or speak with their supervisors. As in civilian medicine, the patients may be vague or evasive in answering your questions for various reasons. You may be surprised to discover that in the military, this is often because soldiers want to return to their mission unimpeded by medical restrictions. This is particularly true of aviators, special operators, infantrymen, and other highly motivated soldiers. It is important to remind them that you are an officer and your medical instructions are orders, and they are required to follow your instructions. If you have any doubts about how compliant a soldier-patient will be, you should speak to his or her supervisor.

In general, your patients will be soldiers in the unit to which you are assigned. It is not unusual, however, that you will also treat soldiers of other units, other branches, and sometimes servicemembers from other countries. It is a good idea to plan in advance so that you have translators or translation tools at your disposal. Useful resources are listed on the Defense Language Institute Foreign Language Center website (*www.dliflc.edu*) and *www.kwikpoint.com*.

Traditional and Nontraditional Patients in the US Armed Forces

Up until recent years, the traditional patients seen by Army doctors have been very fit eighteen- to twenty-five-year-old soldiers who present with illnesses, orthopedic injuries, or battle wounds. In today's Army, however, soldiers may be much older (the current maximum enlistment age is forty-two), heavier, and may have medical issues that were either waivered at induction or developed afterward. Thus medical officers must now be prepared to treat a variety of internal medicine conditions in the field. This means that you must order a large variety of medications to include in your armament of pharmaceuticals, in addition to as many quick lab tests as you or your lab tech can reasonably accommodate.

Another nontraditional addition to the battlefield is the female soldier. Women have demonstrated their value in virtually all roles in the Army and are now eligible for combat roles. As medical providers, you must take their needs into account. Currently, most of the medical equipment sets do not include gynecology textbooks, exam tables, speculums, speculum lights, or any of the other equipment necessary to deliver care to female soldiers. Many MTFs are arranged as open bays that are inappropriate for gynecological care. You need to prepare yourself and your facility for the needs, both acute and preventive, of your female soldiers.

Special Subpopulations: Aviators, Divers, and Special Operators

Certain subpopulations of patients—aviators, divers, and special operators—perform specialized and critical roles in the military and operate in unusual environments. Their needs and treatments therefore often differ from those for the general population of patients.

Aviators are prohibited from flying if they are ill or injured until they are cleared by a flight surgeon or aeromedical PA. Medications that seem benign to the normal population are often prohibited for use in aviators because the seemingly minor side effects can have disastrous effects on the patient's performance in the aircraft. Anything that affects balance, vision, coordination, energy level, alertness, urination, pain perception, or cognition can affect the ability of the aviator to fly safely and can jeopardize the mission and the lives of the whole crew. The same is true for minor injuries or illnesses. A stuffy nose at sea level becomes incapacitating pain at altitude, and a sprained finger can prevent a pilot from pushing buttons. All aviators who seek medical help must be grounded both verbally and in writing, using DA Form 4186, Medical Recommendation for Flying Duty, pending review by the flight surgeon. It is up to the aviator to secure the flight surgeon's review. Though it is not required, it is good form to contact the aviator's commander immediately to notify him or her of your care.

Aviators love to fly and dread visits to the doctor because they are afraid of being grounded. Sometimes they will go to medical providers who are not flight surgeons in hopes that these providers will not know that they have the authority and obligation to ground the aviators. The way to deal with this issue is to immediately contact an Army flight surgeon or aeromedical PA and discuss the case with him or her so that the aviator can be cleared for flight as soon as possible, perhaps even immediately.

Divers have issues similar to those of aviators, though their working conditions are different. Extremes of pressure and temperature, as well as tremendous physical and mental demands, make their jobs extremely dangerous. Thus any care for them must take this into account, and such patients should be barred from returning to work pending review by their dive medical officer (DMO).

Special operators, such as members of the Special Forces, Navy SEALs, or Air Force Pararescue Jumpers (PJs), are completely different from all other patients. You are unlikely to see them because they typically have their own medical support. In the event that you do, however, be aware that they do not operate by the same rules as everyone else. Typically a special operator will present with his or her own highly trained medic, who is there to obtain medical guidance. When you treat special operators, keep in mind that they are intensely mission-focused and will most likely go ahead with their assignment no matter what you say, even if it will kill them. Keep your advice and treatments practical, and tailor your treatments to help them to do their jobs and keep them alive and healthy. If the medicines you prescribe may have side effects, make sure they know about them so they can adjust if necessary. Assume that they will be unable to follow up with you, and dispense to them all of the medications and supplies they will need until they can go to another clinic for follow-up.

Other Patients: Enemy Prisoners of War, Civilians on the Battlefield, and VIPs

Enemy prisoners of war (EPWs) may arrive at your MTF restrained, blindfolded, and guarded. You are obligated, both legally and ethically, to treat them to the same standards as your other patients. You are not permitted to interrogate them or to administer any medications to aid in interrogation. It is extremely important that you monitor your staff's behavior, as emotions may run high in these situations, and you cannot permit them to mistreat or fail to treat the prisoners.

Civilians on the battlefield (COBs) may be brought to your facility by their relatives or by soldiers. You must be prepared for this eventuality by knowing the MEDROE and your commander's opinions on the matter, also known as "the commander's intent." Ethically, you must treat any civilian who was injured or made ill by the activities of the Army. The lines are not always clear, however, and you may be presented with situations where medical ethics run counter to the current regulations. In situations like this, it is very important that you have an understanding of the mission overall and that you and the commander are in close communication so that he or she backs any decisions you make.

VIPs in the form of US military officers or politicians or officers from other countries may visit your MTF for treatment or to tour the facility. Your behavior and that of your staff will be under intense scrutiny during these visits and can influence the mission. Whether you are treating the VIPs or serving as a tour guide, be aware that they are observing your care of your other patients as well. Be respectful, be professional, address them by rank, and don't neglect your other patients. If the VIP is a general—of any branch or country—call your staff to attention when he or she enters the room. It is a gesture that speaks to your alertness, your professionalism as an Army officer, and the professionalism of your staff.

PERSONAL SAFETY AND SECURITY

Don't assume that everyone loves doctors. When you are in uniform, you are an Army officer first. Enemies of the US government see you as an Army officer and probably don't care that you are a physician or a medical provider. If they do care, it may be because they feel that you are more valuable to them as a target of assassination or kidnapping. Unfortunately, there have been many examples of medical providers being targeted in Afghanistan. Because the noncombatant status of Army medics and physicians was generally ignored by the enemy in the Pacific Theater of World War II, the subsequent Fourth Geneva Convention permitted medical providers to carry weapons for self-defense and defense of their patients. All Army medical providers are therefore issued a defensive weapon—a rifle or pistol—and are trained in its use.

Army medical providers must follow the same security precautions as all soldiers in the field. Don't salute or respond to salutes in the field, foreign environment, or civilian environment. Snipers can identify higher-value targets by seeing who salutes whom. That's why you may hear experienced soldiers referring to saluting in the field as "checking for snipers."

When traveling as an individual on military orders, you have the option of traveling in either the Army Service Uniform or the Army Combat Uniform (ASU or ACU). Some soldiers prefer to travel in civilian attire because they feel that a lower visual profile makes them less obvious targets. This is quite sensible when traveling in areas outside the United States that might be hostile to the US military. When traveling within the United States, the risk is lower, and the presence of a US military officer in uniform often is a morale booster and a show of strength for fellow citizens. Nonetheless, don't always assume that someone who approaches you or offers you a free ride has friendly intentions. Travel in groups and be aware of your surroundings.

When in a foreign country, don't advertise your association with the United States. If issued a weapon, keep it with you and secured unless you are within a secure American compound, in which case it must be secured and locked up. Don't venture outside the compound alone.

5

The Army Medical System

This chapter focuses on basic administration within military treatment facilities (MTFs). If you are a full-time medical provider, you will use some of the computer systems described below on a regular basis. If you are a Reservist, you will rarely use them unless you are deployed, but you should still be familiar with them because they will be used by your support staff. An understanding of military health insurance is also very important for both full-time and Reserve medical providers, though for different reasons, as explained below.

MILITARY HEALTH INSURANCE AND ACCESS TO MEDICAL CARE

TRICARE is the name of the health insurance system available to military personnel. More accurately called an entitlement, TRICARE is a system that is available exclusively to active, Reserve, and retired servicemembers and their dependents as a benefit of their service to the country.

All active-duty servicemembers are automatically covered by TRICARE Standard and are provided care at military medical facilities at no charge. If they receive medical care outside an MTF because they have an emergency or are on leave, they must pay a deductible and a percentage of the civilian hospital bill. Spouses, domestic partners, and children of active-duty servicemembers also are automatically covered by TRICARE Standard, charged a small deductible when they receive medical services, and scheduled on a space-available basis. For an extra annual fee, servicemembers and their dependents can purchase TRICARE Prime for themselves and their dependents, which entitles them to pay no deductibles and receive medical care at a higher priority level than if they opt for basic TRICARE Standard. Retired servicemembers and Reservists are eligible for TRICARE as well but must apply for it.

An advantage to working at a military treatment facility is the relative lack of insurance issues. MTFs have medical billers on staff, so the medical provider does not have to be concerned directly with ICD-9 codes. Nevertheless, full-time medical providers need to know the ins and outs of TRICARE because they may encounter patients who are not aware of the health entitlements available to their families, and family health problems can affect soldier readiness.

Reserve and National Guard soldiers are also entitled to free medical care at military MTFs if they become ill or are injured while on duty. They are eligible for TRICARE as well but must pay a nominal fee for themselves and any dependents. Reserve medical providers frequently encounter soldiers during weekend drill who have medical issues or family members with medical issues but have no health insurance. These soldiers are either unaware of the availability of TRICARE or simply make the poor decision to spend the money on other things. It is the responsibility of the medical provider to inform young soldiers that the money they spend on tobacco products and car modification could be more wisely spent on TRICARE. If a Reserve or National Guard soldier approaches you with a medical problem while both you and the servicemember are on weekend drill duty, you are not permitted to provide medical treatment except to preserve "life, limb, or eyesight." Instead, he or she is to be transported to the nearest military MTF via military vehicle or to a civilian facility via ambulance. As a medical officer in a Reserve unit or as a full-time medical officer taking care of Reservists, it is your ethical responsibility to strongly encourage the soldiers to enroll in TRICARE so that even while not on duty, they can obtain medical care for themselves and their families and thus remain fit for duty.

COMPUTERIZED MEDICAL AND DEMOGRAPHIC DATABASES
Defense Enrollment Eligibility Reporting System/Realtime Automated Personnel Identification System (DEERS/RAPIDS)
The Defense Enrollment Eligibility Reporting System (DEERS) is a computer database that lists the names of all active-duty, Reserve, and retired servicemembers and their dependents, as well as DoD contractors and DoD civilians who are eligible for common access cards (CACs or military IDs). DEERS not only lists eligibility for a CAC, but also is used to locate emergency contacts, spouses, and next of kin, and links together TRICARE health entitlements, Servicemembers' Group Life Insurance (SGLI) benefits, and death benefits for funeral and burial. The DEERS database is accessed via the Realtime Automated Personnel Identification System (RAPIDS), generally by human resources personnel.

Medical Operational Data System (MODS)
Medical Operational Data System (MODS) is a system developed by AMEDD to combine several independent computer tracking systems

into one dashboard, allowing commanders and their staffs to track, train, and maintain the health of their troops throughout their Army life cycle. MODS allows users to look at soldiers' medical records, psychological evaluations and screenings, injuries and disabilities, and training status. MEDPROS is one of the components of MODS.

Medical Protection System (MEDPROS)
The Medical Protection System (MEDPROS) is a database that stores information pertinent to the medical deployability of a soldier. Vaccinations, dental exams, psychological assessments and self-assessments, vision, injuries, and disabilities are found here. The information in MEDPROS is accessible to every soldier via his or her Army Knowledge Online (AKO) account, but it can be updated only by AMEDD soldiers who have been granted special permission and have gone through training. (AKO is the homepage for Army members and gives access to Army mail, personnel files, limited medical records, educational records, and much more.)

Dental Classification System (DENCLASS)
The Dental Classification System (DENCLASS) is the software used by the Dental Corps to document and track the dental health of soldiers. It contains the notes from physical exams, X-rays, and procedure notes. It is tied into MEDPROS and is tracked as a component of the soldier readiness system.

Periodic Health Assessment (PHA)
Every year, soldiers fill out the Periodic Health Assessment (PHA), a questionnaire about significant medical events from the previous year. A medical provider evaluates the PHA and follows it up with a physical exam if appropriate. The PHA has replaced the five-year retention physical and is intended to maintain a higher level of deployment readiness among soldiers. PHAs are filled out by all soldiers annually on the computer, and the results are reviewed with the soldier at an annual Soldier Readiness Program (SRP) weekend.

Post-Deployment Health Assessment (PDHA)
A Post-Deployment Health Assessment (PDHA) is performed immediately upon return of a soldier from a deployment, before that soldier is released from deployment orders. Soldiers are understandably eager to be released from their deployment orders so that they can return to civilian life and to their families, and as a result, some may feel motivated to lie about medical issues on their screening forms and when questioned by medical providers for fear that they will be kept on duty and not

allowed to visit their families. These soldiers erroneously believe that they can simply show up at a VA hospital and receive medical care for their issues at a later date. The fact is that they must report any medical issues during the PDHA process in order to establish that their illnesses or injuries happened while on deployment, and therefore are service-connected and thus eligible for VA medical service. Explain to these soldiers and their commanders that they will indeed be kept on orders for a short period, but they can be put on immediate family leave so that they can go home and have their well-deserved reunion.

Post-Deployment Health Reassessment (PDHRA)
The Post-Deployment Health Reassessment (PDHRA) is a question-naire designed to follow up on soldiers who are six months out from their deployments to screen for medical and mental health issues that may have been missed in the PDHA screening or emerged since then.

ELECTRONIC MEDICAL RECORDS
The military and US Department of Veterans Affairs (VA) have led the way in converting medical records over to electronic format. As with most new technologies, the initial efforts were complicated by different approaches to the issue, and thus a number of different electronic medical record (EMR) systems are currently being used. Until recently, the Army's different departmental EMR systems did not interface with one another or with that of the VA. That is now being addressed, and the plan is for all of the systems to be interactive with one another within the next few years.

Inpatient Care
Essentris EMR
CliniComp's Essentris EMR is the electronic medical record system currently being used to document inpatient medical care for 9.6 million servicemembers in the military's fifty-nine hospitals worldwide and more than thirty VA hospitals. Work is under way to integrate this system with those used by the rest of the VA hospitals (VistA) and the Army outpatient facilities (AHLTA).

Composite Health Care System (CHCS)
The Composite Health Care System (CHCS) has been used by the US military since 1988 and allows integration of all the portions of a patient's electronic medical record (stored in the clinical data repository, or CDR), including radiological images, lab values, pharmacy information, dietetics, nursing and medical notes, past medical history, and patient scheduling and demographics.

Armed Forces Health Longitudinal Technology Application (AHLTA)
Medical providers use a module called the Armed Forces Health Longitudinal Technology Application (AHLTA) to interact with CHCS to enter
orders, review lab results, review care and past medical history and demographics, and enter notes. AHLTA-Tactical (AHLTA-T) is a version of
AHLTA that is used in combat support MTFs and by combat medical
providers. The name of the interface with AHLTA-T is Medical Communications for Combat Casualty Care (MC4). MC4 is unique in that it can
operate on a stand-alone computer or cluster of networked computers and
store EMRs until they can be uploaded to the central CHCS database.
MC4 can also collect data from handheld computers used by medics in
the field via an application called AHLTA-Mobile. AHLTA-Warrior
allows providers to access read-only patient data from outside computers.

Tri-Service Automated Cost Engineering Systems (TRACES)
TRACES is the program the Army uses to manage medical inventory.
Having an account allows one to order supplies. Having a TRACES
account, however, requires certification and training, so it is often
assigned to an NCO.

Past Medical Records
Theater Medical Data Store (TMDS)
The Theater Medical Data Store (TMDS) is a web-based application
used to view servicemembers' medical treatment information recorded
in the combat zone.

Clinical Data Repository (CDR)
The Clinical Data Repository (CDR) is the database where all servicemembers' electronic medical records are stored. It is updated by TMDS
and CHCS whenever a soldier receives medical care.

Patient Tracking
TRANSCOM (Transportation Command) Regulating and Command
& Control Evacuation System (TRAC2ES)
The TRANSCOM (Transportation Command) Regulating and Command & Control Evacuation System (TRAC2ES) is an application that
allows medical staff to coordinate and monitor patient movement
between medical facilities. In a tactical environment where patients are
rapidly moving between facilities, it is difficult to locate them, track
their progress through the medical echelons, and monitor their medical
status. This system allows a medical provider to pinpoint a patient geo-
graphically, find out where he or she has been and is going, and observe
his or her current medical status.

Joint Theater Trauma Registry (JTTR)
The Joint Theater Trauma Registry (JTTR) is a system used by deployed trauma nurse coordinators to collect data on battlefield injury demographics, care, and outcomes for military and civilian casualties.

VA Hospital Records
Veterans Health Information Storage and Transfer Architecture (VistA)
The Veterans Health Information Storage and Transfer Architecture (VistA) is the electronic health record (EHR) system used for outpatient and inpatient VA hospital encounters. Since more than 60 percent of medical residents rotate through a VA hospital at some point in their training, VistA is the most familiar and widely used EHR system in the United States.

NONMEDICAL INTERNET ACCESS
Reserve Component Automation System (RCAS)
The Reserve Component Automation System (RCAS) is the system used by full-time Reserve soldiers to access the Internet and perform their daily administrative duties.

Non-Classified Internet Protocol Router Network (NIPRNet)
The Non-Classified Internet Protocol Router Network (NIPRNet) is the standard system used in the Army for nonclassified Internet access when deployed. Access to NIPRNet is limited to military and DoD civilian personnel, and there are strict rules about what sites these personnel are permitted to access while browsing. When deployed, soldiers are assigned a NIPRNet email address and are expected to monitor that new address for communication with the chain of command. Attempts to access unauthorized websites, be they commercial, political, or pornographic, will result in revocation of access privileges, which makes the offender effectively unable to perform his or her job. All traffic on the NIPRNet is monitored by security personnel.

Secure Internet Protocol Router Network (SIPRNet)
The Secure Internet Protocol Router Network (SIPRNet) is a separate secure network used for classified communication. It is accessed by separate dedicated computers, which are located in secure areas. Access to these computers requires a secret clearance, and users must sign in and out of a logbook. Reports up the medical chain of command must be sent via the SIPRNet.

PAPER MEDICAL RECORDS

Paper documentation will continue to exist as long as the Army works in environments where computers, printers, and electric generators break down—which is to say, probably forever. As medical officers, we are responsible for maintaining documentation of continuity of care regardless of the circumstances. Ultimately, even if no printed forms are available, you must write a medical note on whatever you can and keep that note until you can transfer it to the appropriate system. In the worst-case scenario, you can write the note in a journal or on a blank piece of paper with the soldier's full name, service number, and date of birth so that it can be transcribed later onto an SF 600 form or directly into an MC4 computer.

It is not unusual for a medical provider to provide "tailgate medicine"—using an impromptu clinic set up on the tailgate of a truck, with only an aid bag of supplies—during an exercise or when deployed. The well-prepared medical provider will have a few SF 600 forms in the aid bag, but if none are available, entries in a field journal will do. It is highly recommended that medical providers print out each of the forms listed below and put them in a folder or binder to be taken along on exercises and deployments. These forms can then be copied when needed. Alternately, you can store them as photographs or PDF files on a smartphone, laptop, or tablet to be printed out or filled out and printed later as necessary.

Basic AMEDD Forms

Following are descriptions of the forms used most frequently by medical providers, and with which every medical officer should be familiar. The regulation that gives specifics about all medical forms is AR 40-66, Medical Record Administration and Healthcare Documentation.

- DD Form 1380, Field Medical Card, is a paper or plasticized paper tag that resembles a luggage tag. It is supposed to be affixed to any patient treated by a medic in the field prior to transporting the soldier to you. The 1380 has basic identifying information about the patient, their injuries, the interventions, and vital signs when they were treated by the medic. This tag is part of the medical record and should not be thrown away. If the patient's clothes are removed for a trauma evaluation, make sure the patient administrator (PAD) is aware so that he or she can take it off the clothes and enter it into the patient's treatment record. Note that this card is sometimes erroneously called a Casualty Feeder Card.

- DA Form 689, Individual Sick Call Slip, is a very useful but often misunderstood form that is supposed to be filled out by the NCO or officer who sends an ill or injured soldier to sick call. On the right side of the form is an area where the officer can write a note to the medical provider about what happened to the soldier. On the right side of the form are spaces where you can write your diagnosis and treatment, the work limitations of the soldier, and when he or she should return to you. You can also write a note to the soldier's higher NCO or officer if you wish to speak to him or her. In short, the DA 689 could be considered a repair ticket; it's an efficient means of communicating with a soldier's CoC in environments where communication and accountability may be difficult. The DA 689 is not a "ticket for treatment," and the fact that a patient does not have one should not be used as an excuse to send him or her away from sick call. If the patient doesn't have a DA 689, you instead must assume that the CoC does not know that the soldier is at your clinic, and thus you should send the soldier back to his or her NCO or officer with a DA 689 completed by you with your contact information on it.
- SF 600, Chronological Record of Medical Care, aka the Medical Note or Progress Note, is the basic medical note form. It has lines on it for a free-form medical note and a space for patient identifying information at the bottom.
- DA Form 2173, Statement of Medical Exam and Duty Status, known as a Line of Duty or LOD, is filled out by the medical provider to give an opinion as to whether a soldier's illness or injury was incurred when the soldier was on duty performing his or her job and whether there were mitigating circumstances such as alcohol or drug intoxication. This form is then passed on to an investigator, who takes the medical opinion into account when further investigating the circumstances of the illness or injury. The investigation will result in a determination about whether the soldier's injury or illness is service related. Service-related medical conditions are eligible for care by specialists inside and outside the Army, disability payments, VA hospital care, and other entitlements. If a soldier acquires a medical condition while on active duty but does not report it to a medical provider to have a DA Form 2173 completed prior to discharge, he or she is not eligible for those entitlements. Soldiers and providers must understand that VA hospitals will not treat illnesses or injuries for which soldiers do not have LODs filed. In short, *the LOD is extremely important for your patients and can have a lasting impact on their lives.*

- SF 558, Emergency Treatment Record, is a very basic form on which to record emergency medical treatment.
- DA Form 2807-1, Report of Medical History, is the standard medical history form. It is partially filled out by the soldier and reviewed and completed by the medical provider.
- DA Form 2808, Report of Physical Exam, is filled out by the medical provider when he or she performs any physical exam for induction, retirement, schools, fitness for duty, or any other reason. Even though a PA may perform the physical exam and fill out the form, it must be signed by a physician. Each type of physical examination has specific requirements and parameters (including the PULHES grading system), which are described in AR 40-501, Standards of Medical Fitness. It is recommended that the new medical officer have AR 40-501 open and ready for reference when performing the first few hundred physicals, until the specifics are known by rote.
- DA Form 3349, Physical Profile, is a statement by a medical provider that a soldier has a physical disability that limits his or her work capacity for a specific period of time. PAs can write profiles that are ninety days in duration, whereas physicians can write six-month profiles. Only the AMEDD Medical Board reviewers can write a permanent profile, which is based on recommendations by specialists and is written only after evaluating a soldier's fitness for duty.
- DA Form 3894, Hospital Report of Death, must be filled out for every patient who dies in your facility or is brought in already deceased. There may be occasions when deceased combatants are taken directly to the morgue or a temporary storage facility, bypassing the MTF. In those cases, medical providers will be called to examine the body and fill out the DA Form 3894 at that location. When examining the body, you are not performing anything more than a certification of death, documenting identifying marks and your opinion as to the obvious cause of death based on a surface examination only. You are neither required nor authorized to do anything more than that, so you should not remove anything from the body or move anything except to look at dog tags or identity cards in pockets. Make sure that someone witnesses you doing the examination. A formal autopsy will be performed at Dover Air Force Base at a later date.
- DA Form 4186, Medical Recommendation for Flying Duty, aka Up Slip or Down Slip, is used by flight surgeons and aeromedical physician assistants (APAs) to document the flying status of aviation personnel. Aviators may not fly without a current Up

Slip signed by a flight surgeon or APA. Any time an aviator seeks medical care, he or she must be grounded, which you do by checking box 11a on Form 4186, until the aviator is cleared by a flight surgeon or APA. In the event that a flight surgeon or APA is not available to examine and treat the aviator, other medical providers may clear aviators for flight if they speak with a flight surgeon on the telephone, present the patient (describe the patient to another medical provider), and obtain a clearance. That conversation and the name of the clearing flight surgeon must be documented on DA Form 4186 as well as on an SF 600, and the aviator should be instructed to seek out a flight surgeon as soon as possible.

- DD Form 1289, Department of Defense Prescription, comes on a pad just like standard prescription forms. The medical provider is required to print or stamp these forms with his or her name, rank, medical degree, and either social security or Drug Enforcement Administration (DEA) number.
- DA Form 2823, Sworn Statement, is not a medical form but is frequently used by military officers to make statements that can be used in investigations. Examples include incident reports, statements in rape investigations, responses to accusations, formal complaints, and disciplinary or counseling statements.

MEDICAL REVIEW BOARDS

When soldiers become seriously ill or injured and there is a question as to whether they will be able to continue to work in their current assignments or at all, the Army convenes medical boards. These boards consider the soldiers' physical condition at present, their prospects of recovering, the timeline of recovery, expected physical disabilities (temporary or permanent), and the physical requirements of their current assignments. Once that information is evaluated, they must decide whether the soldiers can continue in the current assignments with the disabilities, whether they can be reassigned to other positions that can accommodate their disabilities, or whether they must be medically discharged. These boards are convened at either the federal or state level, depending on whether a soldier is full-time active duty or active Reserve.

The Medical Evaluation Board (MEB) is responsible for evaluating the soldier's medical condition as a whole and determining whether under AR 40-501, Standards of Medical Fitness, his or her condition requires immediate medical discharge. This board makes its decisions based on the physical examinations performed by medical officers and documented on DA Forms 2807-1, 2808, and 2173 and SF 600. The

MEB also collects opinions from outside medical providers and experts and has the authority to mandate further examinations. The board can issue a permanent disability rating to a soldier, which will excuse him or her from certain responsibilities and duties, but this will also permanently preclude the servicemember from certain MOSs. If the soldier fails to follow up with medical examinations and provide the MEB with documentation as directed, the case is referred for disciplinary action, and the soldier may be administratively discharged.

The fact that soldiers potentially stand to benefit financially from medical discharges is a strong incentive for them to comply with the required medical evaluations. Still, soldiers often do not comply, either because they don't understand the repercussions of noncompliance or because they have a secondary gain from delaying the process. It is the unit-level medical officer's responsibility to counsel such soldiers so that they fully understand why they need to seek further medical care and address any barriers to doing that. It is not unusual, for example, for Reserve soldiers to be uninsured or unaware that they must give their civilian physicians permission to share their information with the MEB.

The next step for a soldier who has an injury or illness documented by the MEB is the MOS/Medical Review Board (MMRB), which determines whether this condition precludes the servicemember from performing his or her military specialty "to standard."

Finally, the Physical Evaluation Board (PEB) takes the findings of the MEB and MMRB and makes a determination as to whether the soldier is able to continue in his or her current MOS, can function in an alternative MOS, or is unable to perform any Army job to standard and must be medically discharged.

6

Medical Corps and Medical Support Branches

Upon commissioning, Army officers are assigned a rank and an area of concentration (AOC). The AOC defines the role of the individual officer within AMEDD according to his or her training and specialty. AOCs 60–62 are physicians, 63s are dentists, 64s are veterinarians, 65s are medical specialists, 66s are nurses, 67s are members of the Medical Service Corps, and 68s are enlisted specialties. Each AOC is also assigned a letter that designates a subcategory or specialty.

MEDICAL CORPS (60–62)
Although General George Washington ordered the establishment of an organization of battlefield surgeons during the American Revolution, those early physicians were not commissioned officers. Originally, physicians were grouped with other medical personnel under the Hospital Administration, but eventually Army physicians were commissioned as officers and reorganized separately as the Army Medical Corps. Today, when commissioned, Army physicians are categorized into AOCs according to their specialties and assigned according to these specialties within particular military units. The unit may be in a fixed facility or may be a task force that is sent where needed either as a group or as individuals. Many physicians are deployed as individual augmentees to CONUS (Continental US) or OCONUS(Outside Continental US) assignments and temporarily assigned to certain units.

In the full-time Army, a physician is assigned to a unit within a hospital or clinic and practices medicine or medical administration full-time within that facility. When a tactical unit is mobilized, it is assigned an individual augmentee physician, who is pulled from his or her assignment in the fixed facility and sent with the deployed unit. The position in the fixed facility is then backfilled, usually by a physician in the Army Reserves.

Physicians in the National Guard are often assigned to MEDCOM units and are assigned as necessary and when they are available to perform drill. They are offered missions and deployments as the need arises.

Army surgeons in the full-time Army can expect to be assigned to surgical departments within treatment facilities. Likewise, psychiatrists, ophthalmologists, and a handful of other specialists will be assigned to specific locations. All other physicians, however, can be assigned to administrative or command roles or to general medicine roles as the mission dictates. It is not unusual to see mobilized Army National Guard pediatricians performing sick call duty for soldiers, or a pulmonologist commanding a combat support hospital (CSH). This wide variety of assignments is one of the appeals of Army medicine for many physicians. Army physicians wear the simple caduceus.

MEDICAL SPECIALIST CORPS (65A–D)

The Medical Specialist Corps is composed of physician assistants, occupational therapists, physical therapists, and nutritionists.

Physician Assistants (65D)

Physician assistants enjoy considerably more autonomy in the Army than in the civilian world. When deployed, PAs are expected to perform as general medical officers as independently as possible, seeking guidance as appropriate from whatever physician is available. It is not unusual for PAs to be deployed to clinics or forward bases to run MTFs and supervise combat medics. PAs can be promoted to the level of full colonel and can command medical units.

PAs who are trained in emergency medicine or orthopedics can become certified as Army orthopedic or emergency medicine PAs (65DM1 and 65DM2) and thus eligible for extra pay and bonuses. Further, PAs can train to become aeromedical medicine PAs (flight surgeon 65DM3) or dive medicine PAs (65DM7).

Occupational Therapists (65A) and Physical Therapists (65B)

Physical and occupational therapy were incorporated into the US Army in 1918 in an effort to help the legions of grievously wounded soldiers returning from the battlefields of World War I. Today, as then, Physical therapists (PTs) and occupational therapists (OTs) work with soldiers who have been wounded in action and have injuries such as burns, amputations, traumatic brain injuries, or other conditions to help them regain sufficient function to at least care for themselves and at best return to the fight. PTs and OTs work in a variety of settings, from CONUS healthcare facilities to forward special operations bases. They are commissioned officers and can be assigned to a variety of roles in addition to their field of specialty. Army medicine is mostly occupational medicine, and the goal of returning soldiers to the fight is much better achieved when physicians and PAs work with their PT and OT counterparts to achieve that goal.

Nutritionists (65C)

It has been said that "the Army marches on its stomach." General George Washington was certainly aware of this and took measures early on to establish the Commissary Department to ensure that his troops were well nourished with rations of peas, beans, milk, sauerkraut, cider, fresh vegetables, and beer. Unfortunately, the reality of the day was that logistical problems prevented soldiers from receiving the foods that they were promised, and malnutrition was common. Concerns about soldier malnutrition led Napoleon Bonaparte to offer a substantial reward to anyone who could develop a system to preserve foods for his soldiers. The result was the development of food preserved in jars and tin cans. The Army's experiences in the Civil War and World War I led it to establish the Division of Food and Nutrition to formally study and address the problems of field nutrition in 1917. The results were the development of prepackaged canned and dried field rations, well known to soldiers up until the first Gulf War, and the Meals Ready to Eat (MREs) known to soldiers today.

The American Institute of Nutrition was established by an Army officer in 1928, and with it was born the profession of registered nutritionist. Currently, Army nutritionists develop food and hydration guidelines based on mission, environment, and available foods. They conduct comprehensive nutrition assessments of wounded soldiers, evaluate menus of contract food providers, provide guidance for recovery, and recommend foods and supplements during sustained operations.

NURSE CORPS (66B–P)

Nursing in the military is traditionally traced back to the activities of Florence Nightingale and Mary Seacole in the Crimean War and Clara Barton in the US Civil War. The US Army Nurse Corps was established in 1901, and by World War I, twenty thousand registered nurses were commissioned. By the conclusion of World War II, more than fifty-four thousand nurses had served in the Army, and by then they had become an irreplaceable component of the Army medical system. The current surgeon general of the US Army is a nurse.

DENTAL CORPS (63A–R)

Until the end of the Civil War, the US Army required only that soldiers had sufficient teeth to bite the end off a paper gunpowder cartridge. Not until 1901 did the Army contract with a dental surgeon to provide dental services, and in 1911 it commissioned the first dental officer. The value of field dentists was finally recognized, and by World War I, more than four thousand were commissioned. By the end of World War II, more than fifteen thousand dentists were fielded. DENCOM is now a major command, and for the past decade, dentists have served as commanders of field hospitals, the AMEDD Medical Department and School, and as deputy surgeons general (see "History of the United States Dental Corps." Edited for the Office of the Chief of US Army Dental Corps, May 2011, Jeking). Dentists are generally fielded as far forward as ASMCs and FSMCs, and they are able to perform everything from preventive and repair procedures to damage control emergency procedures, stabilizing patients for transport to higher-level facilities. Dentists are also fully trained as leaders and administrators, and they are valuable assets in mass casualty (MASCAL) situations, able to triage patients and provide first aid alongside medical personnel.

VETERINARY CORPS (64A–Z)

Established in 1911 to care for horses and war dogs, the Veterinarian Corps now employs seven hundred doctor of veterinary medicine (DVM) commissioned officers, eighty warrant officers, and eighteen hundred enlisted soldiers. Veterinarian officers and vet techs provide medical care for military working dogs, ceremonial horses, working animals of the Department of Homeland Security, and pets owned by servicemembers. They provide animal vector control in military areas of operations and care for civilians' pets and livestock in military and civil affairs operations. The Veterinarian Corps is also responsible for food inspection services.

MEDICAL SERVICE CORPS (67–73A–Z)

Medical Service Corps (MSC) officers and soldiers perform the clinical, scientific, administrative, and leadership functions essential to the efficient and effective accomplishment of the Army's health services missions. MSC officers provide invaluable services to the Medical Corps, with administrative and logistical support that helps MTFs function. In addition to administrators, the MSC includes optometrists, podiatrists, pharmacists, psychologists, microbiologists, preventive medicine specialists, biochemists, entomologists, patient evacuation specialists, and lab science specialists.

Unfortunately, there is a history of enmity between the Medical Corps and Medical Service Corps administrative officers. Members of the former are often stereotyped as emotional prima donnas, and the latter as administrative martinets. As with most stereotypes, one can find examples, but in general, it is untrue and the perpetuation of infighting is destructive. The best-functioning medical teams are made up of providers and administrators who are aware of each other's needs, are nondogmatic, and are focused on getting the overall mission accomplished.

Medical Operations Officer (70H) and Medical Supply Officer (70K)
The medical operations officers and medical supply officers are the backbone of the Medical Service Corps. Usually assigned to the headquarters section of a medical clinic, CSH, or MEDCOM headquarters, they are responsible to their commanders for setting up, equipping, supplying, and operating medical facilities.

Psychologist (Clinical Psychologist, Combat Stress Team Member, Aviation Psychologist) (73B)
Of all of the MSC specialties, the psychologists warrant particular discussion. Army psychologists are different from civilian psychologists in that they receive training so that they can operate in non-traditional settings and deliver care that is unique to a war setting. While Army clinical psychologists in the CONUS setting operate much as their civilian counterparts, those assigned to combat stress teams have a different goal: to return soldiers to the fight as quickly as possible. As such, the combat stress team psychologist specifically does not delve into the root causes of soldiers' stress; rather, he or she bolsters soldiers' defense mechanisms to allow them to safely and effectively function on the battlefield, deferring deeper therapy until the soldier can be evacuated if it becomes necessary. The goal of rapidly returning psychologically stressed soldiers to the battlefield is sometimes difficult for newly commissioned medical officers to grasp, but it has proven effective both for the mental health of the soldier and for the functioning of the military, and it is backed by over a century of observations (see *War Psychiatry* by Franklin Jones, MD, ed. Washington, DC: Borden Institute, Dept. of the Army, 1985). Combat stress psychologists are extremely valuable to the medical team and should be used whenever they are available.

ENLISTED MEDICAL CAREER MANAGEMENT FIELDS (68A–Z)
The enlisted soldier with whom most medical providers are immediately familiar is the medic, officially known as a health care specialist (68W). Medics are only one member of a team of enlisted soldiers who are trained in specific medical support skills. Others that you are most

likely to encounter in a medical setting are the patient administrator, or
PAD (68G); the radiology technician, or X-ray tech (68P); the medical
laboratory specialist (68K); and the chief medical NCO (68Z).

NON-AMEDD MEDICAL SUPPORT RESOURCES
The Chaplain Corps
The Chaplain Corps is not part of the AMEDD, but chaplains traditionally have been present wherever medical care is being rendered and are
usually extremely willing to help. Military chaplains are trained in all of
the major religions and are sworn to support soldiers' spiritual needs
regardless of their own personal creeds. Thus, for example, Catholic
chaplains can pray for and with Muslim soldiers, and Jewish chaplains
can pray for and with Buddhist soldiers, in addition to performing services in their own faiths. Chaplains are often valuable for speaking with
soldiers in stress when a psychologist is not available, and they are often
eager to help with triage in mass casualty (MASCAL) situations.

Mortuary Affairs
When a patient dies and you have formally declared and documented
his or her death, your work on that soldier ends, but the work is just
beginning for the Mortuary Affairs and Casualty Reporting Team. Mortuary Affairs is a division of the Quartermaster Corps, the Army command responsible for logistics and supplies, and it operates the morgue
that will receive the body, inventory the deceased's associated belongings, note identifying markings such as tattoos or scars, and package the
body for transport to CONUS. Large MTFs have holding morgues
where the deceased can be held for pickup by Mortuary Affairs. Smaller
facilities will have to designate an area on an as-needed basis. All
remains are flown to Dover AFB in Delaware for autopsy. As a medical
provider, you will occasionally be called to the morgue to assist the
Mortuary Affairs staff by examining a body and filling out a DA Form
3894, Hospital Report of Death.

Casualty Reporting Teams
As soon as a soldier is brought to an MTF, that soldier's CoC has to be
notified, as do various other departments in the military, and finally the
next of kin. These reports are handled by the casualty reporting team
(CRT). If you are approached by a member of the CRT, you are authorized to give the team all of the information requested, as it falls within
HIPAA's military exception clause. You may become overwhelmed
with the number of officers who approach you for information about a
casualty, from that soldier's actual CoC to curious uninvolved soldiers,

but the CRT is the only team authorized to dispense information about the casualty. It is understood that you as the medical provider will speak to the casualty's direct command, but you are not authorized to speak to anyone else. It is unfortunate that rather than finding out about a loved one's injury or death from a uniformed Army officer visiting the home, families often learn of it from Facebook pages, text messages, or other inappropriate sources because medical personnel have shared information with the wrong people. (For more information on the Army Casualty Program, see AR 600-8-1.)

Flight Operations

Many soldiers are transported to MTFs via air ambulance, aka MEDEVAC and "Dustoff" (an alternate name for MEDEVAC helicopters), but MEDEVAC is also authorized to transport medical supplies, ambulatory patients, and medical personnel on a space-available basis. As the medical provider, it is beneficial for you to visit MEDEVAC's flight operations (flight ops) to introduce yourself and to meet the aviators and support staff who transport patients to you. While there, request a tour of the helicopters so you can see the conditions in which the flight medics work and the patients are transported. When you develop a good relationship with the flight ops "battle captains," the ranking officers of the day, you may begin to receive courtesy calls about anticipated patient pickups and offers to transport or pick up supplies. Gaining the trust of the flight crews will also benefit them, especially if they do not have a flight surgeon assigned to them, as they are more likely to come to you when they have medical issues if they trust you.

Aeromedical Evacuation Officer (67J)

A "Juliet" is a MEDEVAC aviator who has undergone additional training in AMEDD doctrine and logistics. This officer is an expert on patient and medical supply movement and is an invaluable asset in a busy theater of operations.

Medical Regulating Officer

The medical regulating officer (MRO) is a corps-level officer who reports directly to the commander (usually a general) of the in-theater MEDCOM. The MRO is responsible for tracking all available patient beds in the major MTFs and coordinating the transportation of all patients within the theater of operations from the point of injury until they are evacuated out of the combat zone. The MRO tracks and directs all flying and rolling vehicles and directs the destinations of the patients they carry. The aeromedical evacuation officer works for the MRO.

Patient Movement Officer

The patient movement officer (PMO) is often an additional duty assigned to a patient administrator within a CSH. This individual, usually a first lieutenant or captain, works with a staff of enlisted soldiers and coordinates with the theater MRO to arrange for patient transport via MEDEVAC (urgent) or fixed-wing or ground ambulance (routine) to higher-level MTFs. The patient movement officer has a very stressful job, as he or she is often caught between physicians, who want their patients moved immediately, and the MRO, who needs to delay some patients' transport because others have been prioritized higher.

MEDICAL BADGES

Badges are insignia worn on the left chest above medals and ribbons. They are indicators of achievements in combat or extra military skills acquired by attending special schools. They can be worn on the Army Combat Uniform as a subdued metal pin-on or sewn-on badge and are worn on the dress uniforms as bright metal insignia.

Flight Surgeon Badges

These badges are awarded to physicians and PAs who successfully complete the six-week Aeromedical Medicine, or Flight Surgeons, Course at Fort Rucker in Alabama. Flight Surgeon and Aeromedical Physician Assistant (APA) Badges are awarded upon graduation, whereas Senior and Master Flight Surgeon Badges are awarded based on flight hours and years of duty.

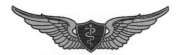

Flight Surgeon   Senior Flight Surgeon

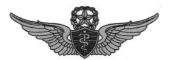

Master Flight Surgeon   Aeromedical Physician
                                Assistant (APA)

Dive Medical Officer Badges

Physicians and PAs who successfully complete the Dive Medical Officer Training Course at the John F. Kennedy Special Warfare Underwater Operations School and Center in Key West, Florida, receive this badge. The Army does not award this badge but permits medical officers to wear the Navy Dive Medical Officer Badge with permission from US Army Human Resources Command.

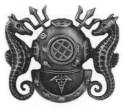

Navy Dive Medical Officer Badge aka "the Bubble Helmet"

Field Medical Badges

Only medics who have served in a combat zone, have treated injuries resulting from combat while attached to a combat arms unit, and have been awarded the Combat Medical Badge can be called combat medics. This distinguishes them from medics who have not seen combat action and those who competed for and were awarded the Expert Field Medical Badge in the noncombat environment. Medical providers are eligible for the Combat Action Badge only if they meet the criteria of treating battle casualties while assigned to a combat arms unit; they are not eligible if assigned to a hospital or aviation unit.

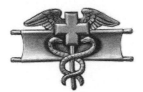

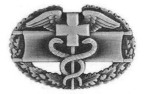

Expert Field Medical Badge   **Combat Medical Badge**

Regimental Crests

A regimental crest is an identifier badge rather than an award. For the medical provider, it identifies the wearer as a member of AMEDD and is worn on the Class A Coat and White Shirt above the right pocket edge, or on the Cardigan or Pullover Sweater on the right chest above the nameplate. Enlisted soldiers wear their regimental crests on the flash of their berets where officers wear their rank.

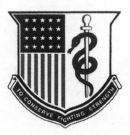

**AMEDD
Regimental Crest**

7

Medical Facilities

The US Army Medical Department has two main missions: caring for combat soldiers on the battlefield and caring for soldiers and their families off the battlefield. In order to fulfill these missions, the Army has medical facilities distributed around the world where large numbers of soldiers are concentrated. In battlefield or temporary environments, the Army field mobile hospitals along with transportation networks move patients to the fixed facilities located off the battlefield. Soldiers who sustain permanent injuries are stabilized in Army fixed facilities and then transferred to the care of the separate VA hospital system.

FIXED FACILITIES
At the time of publication, there are thirty-eight Army medical hospitals and more than seven hundred clinics worldwide that serve Army personnel and their immediate families. Army hospitals are staffed with full-time and Reserve uniformed Army personnel, as well as civilian contractors.

The US Navy operates thirteen CONUS and five OCONUS hospitals, in addition to two hospital ships, and the Air Force operates three CONUS hospitals. Servicemembers can receive care at any of these facilities. Each of the services uses different medical acronyms and supporting documentation, so take care when reviewing medical records from a patient who received care at one of these other facilities.

MOBILE FACILITIES
In addition to their duties in fixed care facilities, Army medical personnel are trained to operate in field medical facilities. Field medical facilities are designed to be mobile and to operate in all kinds of environments and conditions for wartime, relief, or stability missions. The personnel assigned to mobile facilities are trained to rapidly set up the facility and the equipment specific to their departments. The medical staff of a mobile facility is usually augmented by Army

Reservists or by personnel who are temporarily reassigned from their regular jobs in fixed facilities to the mobile facility.

The traditional Army evacuation system refers to each level of care as a "role," (formerly "echelon"), with Role I being closest to point of wounding and Roles III and IV being farthest from the battlefield and more definitive. Note that the role numbering system is the opposite of the civilian trauma levels system. Before reaching a combat support hospital, a wounded or sick soldier will probably pass through two smaller facilities: the battalion aid station (BAS) and the forward or area support medical company (FSMC or ASMC).

Battalion Aid Station (BAS)
The battalion aid station (BAS) is a medical treatment facility (MTF) set up immediately to the rear of the battle lines (if they exist), near the battalion command headquarters. Mobile and austere, it consists of a small tent, an ambulance, a PA or MD, and a team of medics. The BAS provides sick call medicine (ambulatory care) and basic trauma life support (BTLS) and has no holding capabilities. It is considered to be Role I in the Army field medical care and evacuation system.

Forward and Area Support Medical Companies (FSMC and ASMC)
The next higher level of medical care, Role II, is the forward or area support medical company (FSMC or ASMC). These are generally in a more secure area and are set up in larger tents, containers, or fixed buildings. They are staffed with teams of physicians and PAs supported by X-ray, lab, dental, psych, and nursing staff. The FSMC and ASMC are designed to support sick call and occasional trauma for multiple military units in an assembly area or airfield.

Combat Support Hospital (CSH)
A combat support hospital (CSH, pronounced "cash"), when fully configured, is staffed with roughly 600 personnel and is capable of treating and holding up to 256 patients at a time. The facility, which takes roughly a week to set up, consists of rows of tents and containerized operating rooms connected by covered passages located as close to the battlefield as possible but still within a secure area. These container-tent systems are known as Deployable Medical Systems (DEPMEDS). The equipment required for each medical section is packed in hardened plastic or metal containers; these medical equipment sets (MESs) can generally be carried by two soldiers to the designated area and rapidly set up. Although an MES can include hundreds of individual items, each

with its own national stock number (NSN), the whole set also has an NSN so that MESs can be ordered complete from the Class VIII (medical equipment and supplies) warehouse (or resealed when completely inventoried) to expedite rapid mobilization.

The CSH provides the most definitive care a soldier can receive in the theater of operations and is Role III. If the soldier cannot be returned to the battlefield after care at a CSH, he or she is evacuated to a Role IV designated fixed MTF (Landstuhl Regional Medical Center in Germany is a Role IV MTF that receives patients evacuated from the Middle East), and eventually back to CONUS.

SPECIAL MOBILE TEAMS
Forward Surgical Team (FST)
A forward surgical team (FST) consists of four surgeons and sixteen support staff and can operate for seventy-two hours on thirty critical patients before resupply. FSTs are designed to be fully mobile and operational within one hour of arriving at an area of operations. The equipment is packed in containers and can be dropped by parachute onto their area of operations (AO). An FST can operate independently or may be attached to an ASMC or BAS.

Critical Care Air Transport Team (CCATT)
A critical care air transport team (CCATT, pronounced "sea cat") is a three-person team of Air Force medical personnel consisting of a physician, a nurse, and a respiratory therapist. The CCATT can be dispatched to any facility to accompany a patient who requires critical care interventions or monitoring between medical facilities. They carry all of their own equipment and can fly or move the patient in any available aircraft or ground vehicle.

MEDICAL EVACUATION SYSTEM
The military medical evacuation system enables the rapid movement of wounded soldiers from the point of wounding to a location where their wounds can be stabilized, and then subsequently to an operating room where they can be definitively treated. Survival from battle wounds increased dramatically between World War II and the Korean War, from roughly 80 to 90.6 percent, because of the increased speed of evacuation through the use of helicopters. The observed improvement in survivability prompted the development of dedicated, purpose-built MEDEVAC helicopters, called UH-1 Hueys, with flight medics who could deliver medical care while en route to field hospitals. Today the MEDEVAC system uses UH-60 Blackhawk helicopters that fly directly

to the point of injury, often bypassing BASs or ASMCs; medics that deliver advanced trauma stabilization while in flight; and fixed-wing flying intensive care units that carry soldiers from field hospitals to out-of-theater hospitals. Dedicated MEDEVAC units with dozens of pilots and medics are usually co-located with medical facilities and are dispatched by a medical logistical group.

While MEDEVAC refers to the movement of a patient by a dedicated MEDEVAC aircraft, CASEVAC (short for casualty evacuation) refers to the movement of a patient by any available nonmedical vehicle. "Dustoff" is the radio call sign traditionally used by MEDEVAC helicopters because of the way a helicopter dusts off the dirt from the landing zone as it hovers. Every medical provider should take the opportunity to tour a MEDEVAC helicopter in order to appreciate the harshness of the environment in which the flight medics work and casualties travel. The noise inside a Blackhawk helicopter is greater than 106 decibels and makes it impossible to use a stethoscope or hear the patient's words; the vibration breaks most medical equipment; the air blowing through open windows can exceed 125 degrees F or dip below freezing; the helicopter violently pitches and rolls during combat maneuvers; the crew prefers to fly with lights out after dark to reduce attacks (the medic must use night vision goggles to see); and hot metal shell casings may be flying around the cabin if the crew is firing defensive weapons out the windows. In addition, a single flight medic may be treating up to four patients at a time.

When you receive a patient who has been transported by MEDEVAC, consider the additional stress he or she has endured on top of the initial injury, as well as the risk undertaken by the flight medic and three other crewmembers in transporting the patient. Keep these factors in mind too when you consider sending a nonurgent patient to another facility via MEDEVAC: is the test so important that it is worth risking injury or death to the patient and crew?

A Typical Evacuation from the Field
Here's an example of a typical evacuation. After being shot through the leg in a firefight, Private Ryan Jones receives immediate first aid from a combat medic. The MEDEVAC helicopter is thirty minutes away, so the medic transports Jones to the BAS to receive basic trauma life support (BTLS) care and await evacuation. When the chopper arrives, the flight medic takes over Jones's care, loads him onto the bird, and begins transport to the CSH. En route, the flight medic reports to the pilot that Jones's condition is becoming unstable. They decide to land at the ASMC so that the FST there can stabilize the patient. A few hours later,

when Private Jones comes out of the operating room and is loaded onto the bird to continue his evac to the CSH, two more patients that had come to the ASMC for medical problems are loaded with him. The chopper lifts off with the three patients and continues to the CSH. At the CSH, Jones undergoes several surgeries to save his leg, but he ultimately loses a foot and suffers medical issues as well. He is evacuated via fixed-wing MEDEVAC with a CCATT and forty other patients (who are triaged at each stop) to Landstuhl Regional Medical Center in Germany, and then to Walter Reed Medical Center in CONUS. The other two patients who were treated at the CSH are returned to their units on nonmedical transport.

8

Overseas Duty

Overseas deployment is an important event in a medical officer's career. Although some officers are never deployed, it is unusual in today's Army. Failure to perform a deployment is regarded suspiciously by promotion boards and colleagues alike, causing speculation about an officer's incompetence or unwillingness to step up and assume responsibilities.

These assignments do represent some hardship, as they require separation from family and a degree of risk, but compared with those of nonmedical soldiers, medical deployments are relatively easy. Full-time medical officers' deployments can be for a year or longer. Reserve officers' deployments are limited to ninety days for physicians and dentists and six months for physician assistants.

You may see the expression "90 days BOG." BOG is an acronym for "Boots on Ground" and refers to the time spent in the combat zone, as opposed to noncombat training or predeployment areas. References to 90- and 180-day medical BOGs are not actually correct, since the regulation that sets the time limit on these deployments specifies that the deployment and training time must be included in the 90- or 180-day limit.

If deployed with a unit, the full-time Army medical officer (FTMO; this is not an official acronym but will be used in this chapter for simplicity) receives orders, goes to predeployment training, travels to the mission area of operations (AO), performs the mission, and then redeploys home with that unit. The 75 percent of medical officers in the Army that are Reservists, and thus perform shorter missions, rotate into and out of deployed units in short cycles and are referred to as individual mobilization augmentees (IMAs). A deployed unit will host a sequence of 90- or 180-day IMAs that rotate through the positions. In order to accommodate the shorter deployment period, classes of IMAs undergo an abbreviated deployment process at the CONUS Replacement Center (CRC) at Fort Benning, Georgia. Detailed information about CRC, including packing lists, documents, reporting times, and curriculum, can be found at *www.benning.army.mil/infantry/197th/ CRC*.

ORDERS

Once you have been notified that you are being deployed, official orders will be emailed to you shortly thereafter. Official orders are of critical importance, and you must print them out and carry them with you at all times when you are on duty, as they are a legal document authorizing everything you do for the duration of your deployment. Many soldiers keep folded copies of their orders in their hats. You will be required to present orders when you are processed at the CRC and at every stop along your way to your assigned duty station. Copies of your orders should be provided to employers, attorneys, mortgage companies, creditors, banks, utilities, and anyone else who needs to know where you will be during your assignment.

Your orders will list the duration and location of your deployment, plus a lot of information about duty status, pay, authorization for travel, storage of household goods, and many other details. Your orders may or may not include the name of the unit to which you will be assigned or the person to whom you are to report. If not, contact the person who sent the orders and request a deployment memo with information about the unit to which you will be assigned and contact information for the individuals to whom you will report and whom you will be replacing.

CONTACTING THE RECEIVING UNIT

Once you have found out the unit and person you will be reporting to and the person you will replace, contact them via military email (Army Knowledge Online, or AKO). It is good form to introduce yourself well in advance of your arrival, as it reassures the receiving unit that you are en route and gives them plenty of time to arrange for transportation and living quarters. It also gives you an opportunity to obtain information about your assignment. You need to know specifics about the mission you will be performing, and you can only get those details from the individuals you are replacing or supporting. Get their phone numbers so you can talk to them directly if possible. Ask about the types of patients you will be seeing and the skills you should review, the equipment you should bring, and the climate and living conditions.

In addition to arranging the logistics of the mission, take this opportunity to learn the chain of command. If you are assigned to a forward base, as opposed to a hospital, as a medical provider you have two chains of command: the tactical CoC and the medical CoC. For example, you may be assigned to the 101st Artillery Unit in Darulaman, Afghanistan, and you will answer to the battalion commander of that

Telemedicine

All deployed providers and independent duty medical technicians working under an authorized Army provider can access and use the Army telemedicine consulting service. Consultations are answered seven days a week, and recommendations are submitted within twenty-four hours. Consult requests are sent out via AKO to medical consultants in all branches of the military: Army, Navy, and Air Force. The coordinator of this system is LTC (Ret.) Chuck Lappan in San Antonio, Texas; contact him at chuck.lappan@us.army.mil or (210) 295-2512.

Requests for consultations should include a patient narrative and the medical question. Photographs of EKGs, X-rays, and lesions may be attached to the email. Do not include any patient identifying information in the consultation request. You can expect answers from several consultants within twenty-four hours of emailing your request to the appropriate consulting service. The email addresses for the various specialty consultations are listed in Appendix D.

For more information, see the online powerpoint at wrair-www.army.mil/documents/tropmed/teleconsultation.pdf.

unit for day-to-day operations and reports, since you are treating his soldiers. Your higher CoC, however, is the brigade surgeon, who reports directly to the general who controls your battalion commander. Your medical CoC determines the theater medical protocols that you follow, tracks patients, and controls medical supplies. The medical CoC also monitors your performance, writes your Officer Evaluation Report (OER), and issues awards if they are merited.

PREDEPLOYMENT TRAINING AND PROCESSING

Regardless of the duration and location of the training, many of the same basic skills are taught to deploying FTMOs and IMAs: security awareness, weapons training, cultural awareness, use of personal protective and environmental gear, self and buddy first aid, combatives (hand-to-hand combat), radio communications, and others. The full-length predeployment training for FTMOs includes days of both briefs and hands-on practice in training areas that include full-size mockups of villages and cities. The five-day predeployment training for IMAs is primarily in the form of PowerPoint briefs.

In addition to tactical training, all deploying soldiers go through soldier readiness processing (SRP), during which they meet with legal, financial, and human resources personnel to update life insurance, wills, and powers of attorney and deal with pay issues. The SRP also includes meetings with medical personnel, who review health issues, perform physicals, administer required immunizations, issue combat eyeglasses, and dispense required medications. If you take prescription medications for a chronic condition, you must either bring a sufficient supply with you or speak with a physician during the SRP so that he or she can arrange for you to receive a supply to take with you, as well as for in-theater mail delivery of refills through the TRICARE Mail Order Pharmacy (TMOP). A separate day is dedicated to issuing uniforms, tactical equipment, and weapons.

TRANSIT CENTER OR LOGISTICS SUPPORT AREA

At the end of the predeployment training process, the deploying unit or IMA class is flown on a chartered aircraft to a transit center or logistics support area (LSA), either LSA Ali-A-Saleem in Kuwait or Manas Air Base/Transit Center in Kyrgyzstan. At the transit center or LSA, all deploying soldiers present their common access cards (CACs), which are military ID badges, to personnel in a receiving facility, who scan the CACs and register each soldier as present. After being "CACed in," the soldier is officially registered as being in a combat zone and the BOG countdown clock starts ticking. Presence in a combat zone entitles soldiers to extra pay and special legal protections and treatment, as well as combat veteran status upon returning to CONUS.

Because the trip to the transit center crosses multiple time zones and soldiers usually arrive in the middle of the night for security reasons, they arrive jetlagged and disoriented. Adding to the confusion, these areas are crowded with overheated, exhausted, and irritated individuals from many branches of the military, milling about dozens of large, identical, and poorly marked tents in the middle of the night. The FTMOs need only follow their group and don't have to worry about the logistics of where to sleep and how to proceed to the next duty station. They simply load onto buses with their unit and are taken to an LSA, where they will spend several days receiving further training and be issued ammunition prior to proceeding to their mission's area of operations.

Medical IMAs have a harder task: they must immediately separate from the rest of the group and be "CACed in" separately and individually. In other words, if you are an IMA, do not give up your CAC to transit personnel who go around collecting them from members of large units so that they can process them all at once. It is important for IMAs to take the initiative to separate from the larger groups and make their own arrangements. If you fail to do this, you will be caught behind the large units and be at the end of the list for quarters and flights. While this may seem egalitarian, it is one situation where officers do not wait for enlisted to go first. The IMA's skills and time are valuable, and you must not waste time in getting to the mission.

As an IMA, after CACing in, you proceed with your gear immediately to the Billeting or Housing Office to procure a place to sleep and a driver with a vehicle, if available, to transport your gear to the tent. After finding a "rack," or bunk, in the assigned tent and dropping off your gear, you then must proceed to the logistics tent to find the liaison officer (LNO) responsible for the country to which you have been assigned. The LNO will contact your receiving unit, notifying it of your impending arrival, and should also help you arrange a seat on an aircraft or ground convoy to take you the rest of the way to your destination. That "help" is variable, however, as LNOs are not always as well informed as they should be. They may contact the PAX terminal, which is a US Air Force passenger terminal, on your behalf and arrange a seat for you, but sometimes they just direct you to the PAX terminal to arrange your own flight, which will be on a space-available, or Space-A, basis (see Appendix B).

If you are assigned to a small operating base, it will take you several flights and several days to get there. Ask someone at the PAX terminal desk about the route he or she recommends. For example, if you are assigned to a forward operating base (FOB) near Kabul, Afghanistan, you will Space-A from Kuwait to Bagram AFB in Afghanistan. From there, you will Space-A again to Kabul International Airport (KIA). From KIA, you will either Space-A or take ground transportation to your assigned base.

IMAs are responsible for transporting and keeping track of all their gear into and out of the theater of operations. It is not unusual to be issued three heavy duffel bags and a rucksack full of gear in addition to personal gear. Moving all of these bags is hard work and keeping track of it is stressful. Some IMAs choose to leave some gear or personal belongings behind in a rented storage locker. Before deciding what to take, do research on the area where you will be working and learn about the weather, and ask the unit you will be joining and the officer you will be replacing for their recommendations as well. Some units supply tactical gear, protective equipment, and weapons when you arrive, which eliminates the need for you to carry all of that gear with you.

ARRIVING IN-COUNTRY

Once you have arrived in-country (though not necessarily at your duty station), you will need to report to your medical chain of command (CoC) and present your Interfacility Credentials Transfer Brief (ICTB), which is your medical credentials packet (see chapter 9 for more details). If you are an FTMO, the LNO for your unit should collect your ICTB and arrange introductions. IMAs must find their medical CoCs on their own and present their credentials and orders. Once you've met the brigade surgeon or a designated representative, you may be scheduled for briefings prior to moving on to your final destination. Since briefings may take several days, you will need to arrange housing again. The Brigade Surgeon's Office may have control of housing for medical personnel, so ask there before going to the Billeting Office.

ASSUMING THE MISSION

If you are assigned to a large MTF with multiple departments and medical providers, assuming the mission is similar to beginning a civilian job: find out who your bosses are and who works for you; learn your duties, schedule, and administrative requirements; and then get to work.

If you are assigned to a more remote location where you are the ranking or only medical officer, your tasks are more complicated. If you are lucky, you are following in the footsteps of another medical provider who has already set up a functioning medical system and has either guided you through it or left instructions. It is possible, however, that you are the first medical provider and therefore have to set everything up, or that your predecessor may have done a less than complete job. Ideally, the previous medical provider stays until you arrive and performs a proper "right seat ride" with you prior to departing (see chapter 10 for more details). This may not happen, in which case you have your work cut out for you. In addition to responsibility for patient care, you will also be responsible for all of the personnel, equipment, medications, buildings, and vehicles required for the mission.

Following is a list of the steps in taking over an MTF:
- Find the senior NCO or lieutenant assigned to you. After introductions, discuss what's been done, what needs to be done, base rules, patient load, threats (tactical and medical), and expectations of one another. If no senior NCO or lieutenant has been assigned to you, approach the base commander and request one. You need someone with rank and ability, preferably a medic or Medical Service Corps (MSC) officer, to run the day-to-day operations and interact with the enlisted so you can focus on patient care.

- Find the written Medical Rules of Eligibility (MEDROE) and have a discussion with your NCO or lieutenant and the base commander. Find out whom you are expected to and allowed to treat based on the MEDROE, the mission of the unit, and the immediate needs of the base.
- Sign a signature card at Class VIII Medical Supply and Pharmacy.
- Sign hand receipts for large or "sensitive" items, such as buildings, vehicles, computers, narcotics safes, and weapons racks. Take possession of the keys and test them.
- Sign hand receipts for communications equipment: cell phone and radios. Establish rules about contacting you; usually the doctor is "Witchdoctor 6" and the NCO in charge (NCOIC) is "Witchdoctor 7." Check that you have frequencies for or the ability to contact base security and the base commander. If you are the only medical provider or one of few, make sure the medics and commander can reach a medical provider for emergencies twenty-four hours a day, seven days a week, outside of sick call hours. Typically, it is a simple issue of the medical provider on duty carrying a radio.
- Sign hand receipts for narcotics and other pharmaceuticals *after counting them.* Start a new narcotics log or page that clearly separates your count from your predecessor's. Medical providers have been relieved of duty for missing narcotics. Also call in all the medics and do an accountability check for their meds and narcotics.
- Meet all the medics and medical support staff, such as X-ray technicians, lab techs, and patient administrators (PADs). Let them know your medical style, how you intend to supervise them, what you will allow them to do, and what you expect them to do.
- Establish rules for weapons in the MTF and have your NCO or lieutenant enforce them. Don't allow soldiers—either medics or patients—to let their weapons lie around unattended. Set a good example. Just because there is a red cross on your building does not mean it is safe from the enemy.
- Visit the motor pool, the tactical operations center (TOC)/ mayor's cell, the dining facility (DFAC) kitchen, the chaplain, contractor headquarters, the beauty/massage shop, the merchants, and the base security commander. Make your base "walk rounds" a regular habit. Knowing that the doc is present is a tremendous morale booster for troops and a reassurance for the headquarters (HQ) staff. Mechanics and DFAC staff often feel left out and neglected despite their importance to the mission.

- Get computer accounts: MC4, TMOP, TMDS, TRACES, NIPR-Net, and SIPRNet. Make sure your NIPRNet account and computer are functional, as well as your MC4 computers. You will need access to a SIPRNet computer, usually found in the HQ/TOC, so that you or your staff with security clearance can file regular medical reports. If you do not have MC4 running, use an organized paper file system until you get the computer system up. Failure to have MC4 running is unacceptable unless you are in an extremely remote and austere environment; if you are in that kind of environment, paper records are required.
- Familiarize yourself with your vehicles.
- Familiarize yourself with the steps involved in evacuating a patient from your base by MEDEVAC.
- Review MASCAL and trauma plans.
- Establish your medical chain of command, and find out how to communicate with them and what reports they expect.
- Set sick call hours; post them and enforce them. The sick call hours should be early enough that soldiers can see you before going out on missions or training and late enough that they can see you upon returning. The non–sick call times can be used for follow-ups, personal time, and administrative tasks.

LIFE ON A BASE
If you have watched *M*A*S*H* or read *Catch-22*, you will have a strange feeling of déjà vu when living on a combat base. Base culture represents the clash between the orderly world of the home garrison and the chaotic Wild West world of the battlefield. It's a culture where senior NCOs vigorously enforce rules designed for peacetime and soldiers flagrantly disregard personal safety and common sense. It's a place where you can get a speeding ticket for going eleven miles an hour, where you are required to wear a fluorescent reflective safety belt over your camouflage, and where soldiers relax from their actual combat missions by playing video games that simulate battle.

    Sometimes there is logic to the madness. Other times there is not. The safety belts and absurdly slow speed limits seem arbitrary and stupid until you consider the fact that soldiers are far more likely to die from being run over than shot while on base. Knowing that, the ten mph speed limits and safety belts make more sense. Enforcement of sock-length and shirt-tucking regulations in the gym with soldiers who are there to work off the stress of seeing their buddies blown up doesn't make much sense . . . except to the senior NCO, who firmly believes that discipline is what holds the Army together. Medical officers often have problems with arbitrary rule enforcement, because as medical providers, they are thinkers who are trained to recognize anomalies and contradictions and then question them. NCOs and nonmedical Army officers are not used to being questioned and don't receive it well.

The important thing is to not "fight in front of the kids." If someone approaches you to correct your uniform or enforce some other rule, don't pull rank or attempt to argue. Ask where the regulation is found so you can research it, and then retreat somewhere to address the problem. If the person corrects you in front of troops in a loud and conspicuous manner, ask the individual to step away from the others and speak to you privately. When you are in private, ask what he or she believes is a violation of regulations, then remind the individual—calmly but firmly—that such behavior in front of the troops is disrespectful and inappropriate, and that just as he or she expects you to follow regulations, you expect him or her to follow customs and courtesies. Do not threaten to go to his or her commander or to sic your own commander on the individual. It's a good idea to let your commander know what happened so that he or she is not surprised if the other party escalates the situation.

When you are in an MTF, your commander establishes the uniform and weapons policies. Once you step outside the MTF compound, usually defined as the area within the blastwalls, you must comply with base policies.

REDEPLOYMENT HOME
Returning home is essentially the reverse of deploying. Full-time medical officers who deployed with their units return home with those units, after handing off their MTFs to "the new guys." When your mission is nearly complete, get your Officer Evaluation Report (OER) done by your medical CoC, and go over the same steps listed above for taking over an MTF with your successor:
- Perform a "right seat ride" for a few days with your replacement.
- Walk him or her around to all of the base leaders and make introductions.
- Call in the medics and introduce them to their new provider.
- Hand over passwords, keys, combinations, and logs.
- Close out and reconcile the narcotics log.
- Show your successor the reports that need to be sent up and what they contain.
- Give him or her your contact information in case of any questions after you leave.

Reserve Component medical officers must return to the transit center via PAX flights, and then to the CRC to return gear and go through briefings before being discharged from active duty. If you are a ninety-day BOG officer, you must report back to your chain of command and the medical commander with whom you met when coming into the country prior to leaving the theater of operations country. The chain of command must issue you a memo or order that allows you to return home and may also wish to conduct an out-brief or after-action review. They may also issue you a DD-214, Discharge from Active Duty; if you do not get it there, it will be done at the CRC. The medical chain of command may submit award nominations prior to your departure.

Transit Center

To get from your base to your medical chain of command and then to the transit center, you must arrange your own transportation unless you know that an officer has done it for you. By the conclusion of your mission, you should have become acquainted with the staff flight operations (flight ops), so they can get you out on a MEDEVAC or other aircraft. You can also travel by ground convoy by making a request with the base mayor.

Upon returning to the transit center, the redeploying officer must immediately check in with the LNO and PAX staff to find out how to manifest for a seat on the weekly flight back to the CRC. There is only one flight per week back to the CRC, with a limited number of seats. If you miss it, there is no other way home apart from waiting a week for the next flight, so you should arrive at the transit center at least two days in advance to manifest.

CRC

Upon returning to the CRC, you will have a three- to five-day schedule of briefings, equipment turn-in, medical exams, and administrative paperwork. No matter how hard you may try to fight it, you will not be allowed to return home until these are complete. The most important document that you must have upon discharge is the DD-214, Discharge from Active Duty, because it documents your active service time and any awards you received. This is important because the DD-214 officially makes you a combat veteran and entitles you to VA benefits. No DD-214, no benefits. Preserve and protect the DD-214, as you will need it on and off for the rest of your life to take advantage of various veterans benefits.

Benefits and Entitlements

Terminal Leave

When you are discharged from the CRC, you are given terminal leave. This refers to paid vacation days that were accrued during your mission. It is called "terminal" because these days are added to the end of your mission rather than being given to you in the middle of your mission, as they would be if you were deployed for a year. You are paid for these days and technically still on duty, so you are entitled to the rights and privileges of a soldier and cannot be required to return to work until they are completed.

Right Arm Patch and Combat Badge

When you complete a combat mission, you are entitled to wear the insignia of the unit with which you were deployed on the right sleeve of your ACU and may wear the enamel color version of the badge on the right pocket of your Class A Uniform.

Priority in School Choices

One of the privileges customarily given to returning combat veterans is priority in their choices of military schools. If you aspire to be a flight surgeon or want to go to Air Assault School, ask for it before you conclude your mission, and you are likely to be given a spot in the first available class.

VA Benefits

Combat veterans are entitled to the services of the US Department of Veterans Affairs (VA; formerly known as the Veterans Administration). You will be briefed at the CRC about all of the services that the VA offers. Many people are eager to go home and are bored and tired during these briefs, so they miss the information that is presented. Don't be that person. The VA offers health services, psychological and social counseling services, employment assistance, tuition assistance, loans, educational programs, and many other services. It is the VA that administers the Post-9/11 GI Bill, which can be used to pay for continuing education and can be transferred to your children to pay for their education. The VA is an incredible institution that offers benefits unavailable to most American citizens, let alone servicemembers of other countries. You earned these benefits, so don't waste them.

READJUSTING TO HOME

Combat deployments change you. Usually the changes are temporary, but not always. Regardless, the changes in the way you process information, perceive things, and behave toward other people will be noticeable to those back home. Your temperament will be different, and your language may be cruder than before. You may find yourself using profanity frequently and speaking in Army jargon. While your families and coworkers may be willing to accommodate your readjustment, you must be aware of these things as well. You must be open to observations about yourself and motivated to readjust to civilian life. You will be briefed at the CRC about the readjustment period, and methods for readapting will be suggested. Pay attention to this advice, as well as to the resources that are offered. The suggestions just might save your job or marriage.

II

Service as an Army Medical Officer

9

Professional Development

MOVING THROUGH THE RANKS

Because of their advanced degrees, physicians, dentists, veterinarians, and PAs are directly commissioned into the Army as officers. Physicians, dentists, and vets who have just graduated are commissioned as captains, and newly graduated PAs are commissioned as second lieutenants. The rank of commissioning can be adjusted upward for specialties and years of experience. For example, an endocrinologist or dentist with twenty years' experience would likely be directly commissioned as a lieutenant colonel.

Promotion in the Medical Corps is simpler than in the rest of the Army. If you perform your job professionally, pass your physical fitness tests, and attend your drills if you are a Reservist, you are eligible to be promoted after the minimum time in grade. After spending two years as a second lieutenant, for example, you will automatically be promoted to first lieutenant.

In the other branches of the Army, however, promotions are extremely competitive and difficult. They are not automatic, and failure to be promoted twice is a career ender, resulting in forced retirement. Medical school and residency are hard, but so are infantry officer training, air assault training, advanced officer training, and multiple deployments. Medical officers must recognize how hard another officer of equal rank from another branch fought for the insignia that he or she is wearing and should show proper respect.

DA Select Promotion

Promotions are handled by the personnel officer (S1) in your unit at the direction of the commander. When you are within six months of your minimum time in grade and are eligible for your next rank, you should approach your S1 and ask for assistance in assembling your promotion packet, which consists of a set of documents that must be sent to the

Ranks and Grades of the US Army

The "Grade System" was imposed in an effort to cross-level the ranking systems of the various services. The "E" stands for enlisted and the "O" stands for officer. The number next to the letter represents the number of times the soldier has been promoted. Using the grade system, it is easy to see that an Army major and a Navy lieutenant commander are both O-4s, and are thus equal in rank and pay.

E-0	Recruit
E-1	Private
E-2	Private
E-3	Private First Class
E-4	Specialist/Corporal
E-5	Sergeant
E-6	Staff Sergeant
E-7	Sergeant First Class
E-8	Master Sergeant/First Sergeant
E-9	Sergeant Major/Command Sergeant Major/Sergeant Major of the Army
O-1	2nd Lieutenant
O-2	1st Lieutenant
O-3	Captain
O-4	Major
O-5	Lieutenant Colonel
O-6	Colonel
O-7	Brigadier General
O-8	Major General
O-9	Lieutenant General
O-10	General

medical specialty Department of the Army Selection Committee (hence DA Select) in Washington, DC. The committee, or promotion board, meets monthly to review the promotion packets for each specialty, branch, and rank, and then announces its selections. The promotion packets are complicated and detailed, so you must work closely with your S1 to ensure that they are complete, correct, and properly submitted. Information about how to fill out Officer Evaluation Report Support Forms and assemble promotion packets, as well as promotion announcements, can be found at *www.hrc.army.mil*.

Unit Vacancy Promotion

An alternate route to a higher rank is a vacancy promotion. In the Army, every unit has a Table of Organization and Equipment (TO&E), which lists personnel positions, or slots, that are necessary for the functioning of a unit. For example, a medical company will have slots for the commander, the executive officer, two physicians, three PAs, four nurses, a mental health worker, and so on. In order to establish a chain of command within the unit, each of the slots is preassigned a rank, and it is expected that the individual occupying that personnel slot will have that rank. If there is a vacant spot in the unit that is designated for a rank higher than that of the available officer, and if that officer is eligible, with sufficient time in rank and proper credentials, higher command may approve a move into the higher-ranked slot and promotion of the officer selected to fill the slot. Medical officers may remain in a TO&E slot even if they have a higher rank until they are two ranks above, at which point they must be moved to another slot or into another unit that has a slot that accommodates their rank.

EVALUATIONS

Officer Evaluation Report (OER)

Every year, with each reassignment, and after every deployment, officers must be evaluated by their immediate supervisors, and each of these evaluations is documented on a DA Form 67-9, Officer Evaluation Report (OER). The OER summarizes your goals and accomplishments, gives your job description, and contains your supervisor's opinions as to your performance and suitability for promotion. You should provide your supervisor with a DA Form 67-9-1, Officer Evaluation Report Support Form (OER Support Form), which you have filled out with your goals, accomplishments, and job description, so that he or she doesn't have to hunt for that information. It is a good idea to ask to see your supervisor's previous OER so that your goals can be consistent with his or hers and those of the unit.

Army Physical Fitness Test (APFT)

Soldiers are required to maintain a high level of physical fitness so that they are deployable at all times. To that end, you are expected to perform regular physical training (PT) individually and as part of a group. On a regular basis, at least every six months, the Army conducts Army Physical Fitness Tests (APFTs) for the official records, as well as diagnostic APFTs to monitor soldiers' progress. The APFT consists of sit-ups, push-ups, and a two-mile run. The minimum number of push-ups and sit-ups and the maximum run time are defined by the soldier's age and are listed on a chart. A minimum passing score is 180, while the perfect or "max" score is 300. Soldiers with physical profiles can be excused from certain events or perform alternative events such as walking. Soldiers who fail the APFT are "flagged" and are ineligible for promotion or schools. For more information, see *www.army-portal.com/ pdf/apft.pdf*, FM 21-20, Physical Fitness Training, and AR 600-8-2, Suspension of Favorable Personal Actions.

DA PHOTO

Every officer is required to have a Department of the Army (DA) photo on file with the Army in a database called the Department of the Army Photo Management Information System (DAPMIS). The DA photo must be taken by a professional photographer contracted by the Army. You are not permitted to have your DA photo taken anywhere else or submit one of your own. Most military installations have facilities where these photos can be taken at no charge and uploaded to your file. Call for an appointment, because they are often busy.

You are responsible for bringing your Class A Uniform (green or blue) and for having your ribbons properly arranged on your chest. Covers (hats) are not worn in Army DA photos so make sure your hair is trimmed or arranged to Army standards (AR 670-1). The photographer will position you correctly and according to regulations but cannot correct your awards. The promotion board looks closely at your uniform and awards in your DA photo and could reject your promotion request if you do not fit Army standards for appearance of professionalism and fitness or if your awards are incorrectly placed. Uniform guidebooks are available at the post exchange (PX) if you prefer to do the research on your own, but it is always a good idea to have someone else look you over; even though items may look straight when you pin them on, they may be crooked or incorrectly placed after you put on the jacket. To make sure you are squared away before going to your appointment at the photography studio, present yourself to a knowledgeable officer or senior NCO who can look over your appearance in uniform.

MEDICAL CREDENTIALS

The Army uses the Centralized Credentials Quality Assurance System (CCQAS, *https://ccqas.csd.disa.mil*) to track medical credentials. When you are appointed as a medical officer, a Provider Credentials File (PCF) is established and uploaded to CCQAS. The PCF must be updated regularly (generally twice a year); this is done by the "Credentialing Officer," who is either a contractor or a Medical Service Corps officer assigned the duty. The Credentialing Officer will contact you once or twice a year and ask you to update your contact information, civilian employment (if you are a reservist), medical licensure, education, Basic Life Support Certification, and Malpractice Information.

When you are assigned to provide patient care outside of your designated unit (or if you are a Reserve Component officer performing medical support for annual training), your medical credentials must be sent to the location where you will be practicing in the form of an Inter-facility Credentials Transfer Brief (ICTB). You will need to fill out several forms (listed below) and submit them to the official responsible for compiling the ICTB—usually the Credentialing Officer. Even though the ICTB is supposed to be transmitted electronically well in advance of your mission, it is a good idea to bring a paper copy of the ICTB with you to your assigned duty station as a backup.

> **FORMS REQUIRED FOR CLINICAL PRIVILEGES**
> You will need to fill out and submit the following forms in order for the ICTB to be completed:
> - DA Form 4691, Initial Application for Clinical Privileges
> - DA Form 5754, Malpractice History and Clinical Privileges Questionnaire
> - DA Form 5440-1–58, Delineation of Clinical Privileges
> - DA Form 5441-1–58, Evaluation of Clinical Privileges

PERSONNEL RECORDS AND STAFF
Interactive Personnel Records Management System (iPERMS)
As you progress in your career in the Army, you will accumulate documents that are pertinent to your career. Annual written reviews (OERs), notifications of promotion, training documents, awards, orders, special assignments, and any other documents all become part of your file. Because the Army, like all organizations, is moving toward electronic record keeping, your paper documents are scanned and entered into records that you can access on the Interactive Personnel Records Management System (iPERMS) website. It is advisable to periodically review your iPERMS record to ensure that your documents have been entered into the electronic record.

Human Resources Command (HRC)
The organization responsible for all human resources or personnel issues in the Army is the Human Resources Command (HRC), formerly

known as Personnel Command (PERSCOM). HRC generally operates in the background for most officers, but its operations are critical to your career. Many of the documents you find in your iPERMS files are generated by HRC. If you have any questions about your career that your direct chain of command cannot address, contact HRC at 888-ARMYHRC (888-276-9472) or askhrc.army@us.army.mil.

Personnel Officer

The personnel or human resources officer in an Army organization is the S1 (or sometimes the G1, if the highest-ranking officer in your unit is a general). The S1 is the officer to whom you should address any questions about pay, promotion, and training. He or she is also the person with whom you should cooperate when addressing health issues in a unit, as the S1 is responsible for tracking soldiers if they go to a healthcare facility and for all of the personnel actions that must take place in the event a soldier is injured or falls ill. Medical records that are generated in your facility are ultimately the responsibility of the S1 of each patient's unit. The S1 may come to you asking for copies of medical records so that he or she can process soldiers' records and adjust their pay, leave, or other issues. S1s are considered to be personnel with need-to-know status under HIPAA and DoD HIPR and are entitled to those records.

AWARDS

Military awards can be given to an individual or to a military unit. Awards are usually presented by commanders to award recipients in a formal manner in front of soldiers assembled in a formation. If you are to be presented with an award, you are called to the front of the formation to face the commander, and you stand at attention while a narrative of your award-worthy actions is read to the assembled troops and audience. The commander then hands you the certificate or pins the award on your uniform, and you are given the framed document and medal presentation box.

Awards appear in five forms: unit commendations, certificates, ribbons, cords, and medals. Ribbons, cords, and medals all have specific requirements associated with them and must be applied for and approved by the appropriate level of command. In general, the more prestigious the award, the higher ranking the officer that must approve it.

Unit commendations are awarded to Army organizations that are recognized for their performance above and beyond others. Each soldier in that unit who was a member at the time of the award is entitled to wear a unit commendation award on his or her uniform.

Certificates are paper documents that are awarded by the local commander to individuals who have performed duties that are notable but do not rise to the level of a cord, ribbon, or medal.

Service ribbons are higher than certificates and are usually awarded in recognition of successful training or missions performed. They are not awards, per se, but rather indicators of achievement. Thus, an officer who completes Officer Basic Training is awarded the Army Service Ribbon (usually the first award any directly commissioned officer wears on his or her uniform).

Cords are worn on the left or right shoulder and are also referred to as aiguillettes or fourragères. They can represent awards given to entire units, such as the Croix de Guerre worn by the 369th Infantry Harlem Hellfighters for service in World War I France. They can also indicate special training or duties; for example, an infantry soldier is awarded a blue cord to wear on the right shoulder upon completion of infantry training, and US presidential aides wear a gold cord on the right shoulder.

Medals can be awarded for valor in battle, for non-combat achievements, or for honorable military service for a prescribed duty (in a particular geographic area or mission). Those that are awarded for valor or achievement are known as "individual decorations," while those awarded for military service are known as "service awards." Individual decorations are considered to be more prestigious as they are visible recognition of service above and beyond expected duties.

While the layman refers to all awards as medals, actual medals are metallic medallions of various shapes dangling from ribbons of specific colors and patterns. Most people never see the full medals, because while it is permitted to wear full-sized medals to formal occasions, most officers opt to wear only the ribbon slider portion of the medal arranged on a "rack" on their left chest alongside their service ribbons. Full-sized medals and ribbons are never mixed. One either wears *only* the full-sized medals, or just the medal ribbon sliders and service ribbons.

However one chooses to wear them, awards are arranged in order of precedence. Individual awards can be augmented with metal "devices" (silver or bronze oak leaves, stars, or letters) that indicate multiple presentations of the same award, meritorious service, or valorous service.

If you are a member of the National Guard, you are also eligible for state awards. These awards are worn only when on state duty; do not wear them if you are on federal duty. All state awards are lower in precedence than federal awards and follow them on the medals rack.

Awards are an extremely sensitive subject with soldiers. Other soldiers or officers who performed the same duties as you may not have

United States Military Decorations

Decorations (in order of precedence)	Awarded for		Awarded to			
			United States Personnel		Foreign Personnel	
	Heroism	Achievement or Service	Military	Civilian	Military	Civilian
Medal of Honor	Combat		War[1]			
Distinguished Service Cross	Combat		War	War[2]	War[1]	War[2]
Defense Distinguished Service Cross		War Peace	War Peace			
Distinguished Service Medal		War Peace	War Peace	War[2]	War Peace	War[2]
Silver Star	Combat		War	War[2]	War	War[2]
Defense Superior Service Medal		War Peace	War Peace			
Legion of Merit		War Peace	War Peace		War[4] Peace[4]	
Distinguished Flying Cross	Combat Noncombat	War Peace[7]	War Peace		War	
Soldier's Medal	Noncombat		War Peace[7]		War Peace[7]	
Bronze Star Medal	Combat[3]	War Peace	War Peace	War Peace	War Peace	War Peace[2]
Purple Heart	Wounds Received in Combat		War Peace[6,7]	War[6,7] Peace[6,7]		
Defense Meritorious Service Medal		Peace	Peace			
Meritorious Service Medal		Peace	Peace		Peace	
Air Medal	Combat[3] Noncombat	War Peace[7]	War Peace[7]	War	War	War
Joint Service Commendation Medal	Combat[3] Noncombat	War Peace	War Peace			
Army Commendation Medal	Combat[3] Noncombat	War Peace	War[5] Peace[5]	War	War[5] Peace[5]	
Joint Service Achievement Medal		Peace	Peace[5]			
Army Achievement Medal		Peace	Peace[5]		Peace[5]	

Notes:
1. The Medal of Honor is awarded only to United States military personnel
2. Only rarely awarded to these personnel
3. Awarded with bronze V device for valor in combat
4. Awarded to foreign military personnel in one of four degrees
5. Not awarded to general officers
6. Awarded to military and civilian personnel wounded by terrorists or while members of a peacekeeping force
7. Approval authority for peacetime award is Headquarters, PERSCOM

been similarly awarded, even though they may have been just as worthy. There may be colleagues who do not think that you deserved the award, even if you did. Awards bring up emotions and can be sources of great pride or resentment. Thus there are certain unwritten rules to which officers should adhere. First, never ask for an award. If you have to ask for it, your service was probably not worthy of recognition. Further, asking for an award suggests that you are a glory seeker or medal chaser, which is considered beneath contempt for an officer. If you feel that you achieved something, there were most likely soldiers beneath you who made it possible. Your job as an officer is to nominate *them* for the appropriate awards.

Wear your awards properly. If you are unsure of the precedence or sequence of your awards, get help from an NCO or fellow officer before putting them on your uniform. Don't put on an award unless your commander presents it to you. Even if you receive the award in the mail because you were attached to another unit, and it was awarded to you after you left, take it to your executive officer so that he or she can give your commander the option of awarding it to you in front of your unit. If you are unsure of whether you are permitted to wear an award, speak with your S1 to see if you have documentation to prove that you are entitled to wear it.

Do not openly question other officers' or soldiers' awards in a public setting. If you have serious doubts about an award, discreetly ask the S1. In general, it is best to steer clear of these issues, as arguments about them can become ugly. That said, good-natured teasing is normal in social settings. If you do decide to teasingly question an award, make sure you know the story about it before saying anything, to avoid embarrassing yourself or your friend and colleague.

Never gloat about an award. No matter what you did to be recognized with the award, there are probably others who were more worthy than you who were not awarded. No matter how proud you or your family may be, show humility when you are awarded. If you are married, it is a good idea to share this rule with your spouse so that he or she avoids uncomfortable situations with the spouses of unawarded officers. If you need examples of this, look to the behavior of Medal of Honor recipients. Most are modest to a fault and reticent to talk about their awards.

Information about specific awards can be found in AR 600-8-22, Military Awards.

TRAINING
It is axiomatic that the life of a doctor, dentist, or veterinarian is a lifetime of training. This is also true of the life of a soldier, as the military life requires constant training to prepare the soldier for battle. Thus it follows that military medical officers are also constantly practicing

medicine, as well as periodically training to learn new or refine old soldiers' skills. Full-time military medical officers have yearly training schedules incorporated into their calendars as part of their regular duties. Reserve Component medical officers are entitled to an annual medical training stipend (currently $2,500), which can be spent on books, seminars, or medical conferences. These activities must be coordinated through Training NCOs, who arrange for your authorization, travel orders, and reimbursement.

Each unit has a Training NCO responsible for making sure that the enlisted soldiers and officers in the unit receive the training they need. The system they use to enroll soldiers into courses is called the Army Training Requirements and Resources System (ATRRS, pronounced "aye-taars"). ATRRS is accessible for individual soldiers (see *www.atrrs.army.mil*), but for Reserve Component soldiers, the Training NCO must first obtain approval for funding.

The required courses for a medical officer are the Basic Officer Leaders Course (BOLC) and Advanced Officer Leadership Course (AOLC), aka Captains Career Course. Participants in the Specialized Training Assistance Program (STRAP) are offered the optional Soldier Focus Readiness Review (SFRR) Course to orient them to the basics of Army life before attending the BOLC.

Basic Officer Leadership Course (BOLC)
Newly commissioned medical officers are expected to take Phases I and II of the Basic Officer Leadership Course (BOLC) as soon as possible after commissioning. Phase I is the correspondence or computer portion of the course. Phase II is the resident portion and takes ten to thirty days, depending on whether the officer is full-time or in the Reserves or National Guard.

In the full-time Army, this is fairly easy, as the officer's schedule is built around training courses. For Reservists, scheduling basic training is more difficult, as it is not permitted to interrupt residency schedules and takes a lower priority than a medical officer's civilian schedule. Members of the Reserves may not have the ability to take the time off from work to attend BOLC immediately and are permitted to attend drill until they can arrange the time to take the course. They simply schedule the course far in advance to accommodate it into their busy schedules. Medical residents are permitted to delay attendance until completion of their residencies but then must take the entire course in order to be promoted, although they may schedule it for vacation time.

Full-time Army officers are required to take the full seven-week course. Reserve officers take the abbreviated Reserve Component (RC) course, which has a correspondence portion and a ten-day field portion. Officers are paid their officer salary to attend training courses, which, depending on whether you are a resident or a full-fledged doctor, could represent either a raise or a dramatic pay cut.

As with most Army medical training, BOLC takes place at Fort Sam Houston in San Antonio, Texas, where officers learn basic soldiering and basic Army administrative skills. During the correspondence and classroom components of BOLC, you learn how to wear your uniform, march, stand in formations, salute, and interact with the enlisted troops and other officers. During the field component of the training, you are taken to Camp Bullis in the hills of San Antonio, where you are taught basic soldiering skills: handling weapons, using a gas mask, taking cover, basic physical fitness training, land navigation, convoy operations, moving patients, and combatives (hand-to-hand combat). While training, the classes are divided into different ranks, but everyone undergoes the same training and is subordinate to the trainers (in other words, a newly commissioned colonel may not refuse to do push-ups or clean a weapon on the basis of rank while attending BOLC).

Medical BOLC is more rugged and strenuous than some civilians are used to, but it is considerably less stressful than what members of the other branches undergo in BOLC. Unlike the regular BOLC, which trains fit twenty-five-year-old first and second lieutenants, the medical BOLC classes are made up of medical professional men and women ranging from twenty-two to fifty-eight years old, some of whom have never done push-ups in their lives. The course directors are dedicated to getting everyone through the course alive and uninjured, but they are also in the business of teaching soldiering skills. It is a good idea to begin a fitness routine at least a month before reporting to camp, emphasizing push-ups, sit-ups, and running (prepare for two miles a day). While attending BOLC, you will make mistakes, get yelled at, have to do things that you feel are beneath you or think you can't do, go days without a shower, and be uncomfortable. But you will have it much easier than the enlisted soldiers that you will lead, and you will survive. Pack plenty of wet wipes, humility, and an extra serving of toughness.

Advanced Officer Leadership Course (AOLC)

The Advanced Officer Leadership Course (AOLC), aka Captains Career Course, is the transition course that teaches junior officers (first and second lieutenants) how to perform as leaders of small units—companies and below—and serve in staff positions. In the nonmedical branches of the Army, this course is required for promotion. In the medical branches, this rule is not as strict. As officers advance through the ranks to O-5 and O-6, the opportunities for promotion become fewer because there are only a limited number of slots for O-6s, so having additional training gives the hopeful candidate an advantage.

Correspondence Courses

Many Army courses involve a correspondence portion. Once you have registered through ATRRS, the correspondence study materials are mailed to you or you are given access to a computer portal. After you've completed these materials, you usually must take an online test, although some courses still mail scanner cards to you. Upon completion of the correspondence portion, you are eligible for the residence portion of the course. The Captains Career Course and the Physician Assistant Emergency Medicine Specialty Course are correspondence courses.

Predeployment Courses

Before deploying on an active-duty mission, medical providers are expected to go through specialized medical training to prepare them for combat medicine. This training is conducted by the Center for Pre-Deployment Medicine (CPDM). Tactical Combat Medical Care (TCMC) should be taken by all physicians and PAs prior to deployment, as it teaches wounding patterns and advanced trauma life support skills. Unfortunately, many Reserve Component Training NCOs and commanders are not aware of these courses, let alone their importance, and they are not usually put on the predeployment task lists for deploying units. Similar courses are offered for nurses and medics.

Postgraduate-Level Courses

For licensed physicians, PAs, veterinarians, and dentists, AMEDD Center and School offers postgraduate-level courses and symposiums. Many of these courses are designed with the active-duty provider in mind, but Reserve Component providers are encouraged to attend. The catalog of courses can be found at *www.cs.amedd.army.mil/ahs.aspx# cpdm*.

Military Medical Specialty Training
Flight Surgeon Course
At the US Army School of Aviation Medicine at Fort Rucker, Alabama, the Flight Surgeon Course trains physicians and PAs to become Army flight surgeons. This six-week course teaches candidates the principles of flight, aviation technology, SERE (survival, escape, rescue), water survival, crash survival, crash investigation, principles of aviation

medicine, and aviation medicine administration. Graduates are qualified to wear flight surgeon wings, provide medical support to aviators, fly as crew aboard Army aircraft, and receive flight pay.

Dive Medical Officer Course
Conducted at the John F. Kennedy School for Special Warfare in Key West, Florida, this is the most physically and mentally challenging course in the Army. Dive medical officer candidates train with Army Special Forces "Green Beret" medics to learn underwater operations using scuba and hard-helmet diving, and then learn underwater physiology, pathology, and care of diving accident patients.

Residency in Aerospace Medicine (RAM) Program
AMEDD offers military medical residents a specialty unique to the military: the Residency in Aerospace Medicine (RAM) program. RAM candidates attend flight medicine school, dive medicine school, and jump school to learn about the physiologic stresses and injuries that accompany these high-risk endeavors. After earning their qualification badges in each specialty, "RAMs" are uniquely prepared to provide medical support to special operations soldiers as their primary care physicians.

Continuing Medical Education
All Reserve Component medical officers are entitled to annual continuing medical education (CME) funds. These funds, usually about $2,500 annually, can be used to fund "any one medical event," which can be anything from a purchase of medical textbooks to attendance at a medical convention. The money is not automatically disbursed, however. The Training NCO must enter the requested CME event into ATRRS in advance of the event and the chain of command must approve it. When approved, you may then attend the event or make the purchase, and then submit a DA Form 1351, Travel Voucher, for reimbursement.

10

New Duty Assignments

INTEGRATING INTO A NEW UNIT

When you join any new unit, your first order of duty is to report to your commander (or to the executive officer for presentation to the commander). It is never good form for a commander to learn about your presence from subordinates, and it is extremely rude to start poking around a unit and asking questions before your formal introduction. Make an appointment if possible, and make sure your uniform is correct and you have orders in hand for presentation. This is a classic first-impression situation. Your new commander's job is to welcome you and show you around or assign someone to do it.

Either at this meeting or at a subsequent one, it is important to discuss your new commander's expectations of you, known as the "commander's intent." This goes beyond your formal job description, which you should have looked up in your orders or in a manual prior to arriving. The commander's intent is your boss's philosophy of how to run the unit and how he or she expects the mission to be executed. The meeting is your opportunity to learn about your new boss's personality, such as whether he or she is a "get-the-job-done" or "by-the-book" person. You should also get an idea of the commander's specific expectations of you and a timeline for those expectations.

In general, when a superior officer speaks to you, get out a book or pad and write down what he or she is telling you. This demonstrates that you hear what the commander is saying and are taking it seriously. You can also use your notes to refer to later.

After you have met your commander and executive officer and have completed your tour, it is time to make your own rounds and meet your colleagues and fellow officers, as well as the troops who answer to you. Start with your immediate subordinates and work your way outward to the soldiers and officers with whom you will be interacting but who are not necessarily in your chain of command. Learn your soldiers' names as soon as possible. At some point during your introductory meetings, you need to make it clear that you have met the commander and are aware of his or her intent and the unit's mission; when you meet the officers, also indicate how you intend to support that mission.

Find out who your patients are going to be and learn your Medical Rules of Eligibility (MEDROE). When nondeployed, you will most likely be working exclusively with soldiers. When performing joint services exercises or during state emergencies or deployments, you could be treating members of other services or even citizens of other countries. If that is the case, you need to prepare yourself and your medical team to accommodate those patients.

There may be deployments where you are the highest-ranking medical officer in the area and have no commander. In this case, find the next-highest-ranking officers in your area of operations, as well as the base commander and OICs of various organizations in your AO, and make your introductions to them. Although they will know that you do not fall under their command, they will appreciate the respect you paid them and will also appreciate it if you ask their opinions about what medical issues you are likely to encounter in their areas of operations.

If you are replacing someone, it is standard for the Army to execute a Relief in Place/Transfer of Authority (RIP/TOA), commonly known as a "right seat ride." During this period, you are expected to shadow the individual you are replacing, as if he or she were still driving and you were the passenger learning the routes and operation of the vehicle. During the latter half of the right seat ride, your predecessor is supposed to observe you while you take over control so that he or she can offer advice. Once the RIP/TOA is completed you have officially "assumed the mission."

REPORTS

Reports are a necessity of military life. You can expect that your higher headquarters is going to want regular reports about the number of patients you have seen, their wounds and disease or nonbattle injuries (DNBIs), demographics, and other details. You will also be asked to provide reports about supplies, patient movement, and various other aspects of your medical operations. Your NCOIC should be able to handle many of these reporting duties, but you are ultimately responsible for them, so you must look over the reports periodically.

It is easy to become irritated about the number of reports required of you, particularly if the reports seem senseless. Keep in mind, however, that though you may not see the utility of reports that contain little information, higher headquarters requires the information to properly distribute supplies and personnel and perform any number of other logistical tasks that may be unknown to you but essential to the mission. Be patient, be diligent, and supply the requested information.

AFTER ACTION REVIEW (AAR)

An After Action Review (AAR) is both a meeting that takes place immediately after a significant military activity and a written report of that meeting. The proper way to conduct an AAR is to gather all individuals who were involved, not just the leaders, and methodically go through the goals of the mission, the actual events of the mission, what was achieved or missed, what could have been done better, what could have been improved, and what went wrong. The meeting should be directed by the highest-ranking person present or a designee, and it should be conducted in a methodical manner so that nothing is missed and everyone who was involved or observed has an opportunity to contribute openly. Minutes are kept so that they can be used as a reference when writing the official report. AARs are the basis for a program called Army Lessons Learned and are designed to be used as a reference so that the Army is continually improving its operations. (For more details on the Lessons Learned programs of the various branches, see the websites given in Appendix D.)

The meeting and report are extremely valuable for a number of reasons. The meeting allows soldiers to vent their concerns in a private and controlled place, and the report lets the writer make recommendations to higher-ups regarding future operations. The reports can also serve as historical documents for future generations. AARs written by Major Dick Winters during World War II are still studied at the US Army War College and were an important historical source for the book and TV miniseries *Band of Brothers*.

MEETINGS

Sometimes higher headquarters likes to have a medical representative at its regular meetings. You may attend or assign a junior MSC officer to represent you and bring back information from those meetings. Communicate with the CoC and find out if they require you specifically or if a representative will be sufficient.

III

Social and Other Matters

11

Benefits Available to
Army Officers

The sacrifices of military life are great. In recognition of this, the nation confers upon servicemembers benefits that are unavailable to the civilian population. Many of these benefits are underutilized because they are unknown. The benefits discussed in this chapter apply to your spouse and children, and unless otherwise stated, they continue even after you have retired from service. Taking advantage of the services listed can save you a significant amount of money and go a long way toward compensating for some of the stresses borne by you and your family. If you are retired, you may be surprised to learn how many resources are available to you. These benefits are not gifts—you earned them.

FINANCIAL BENEFITS
United Services Automobile Association (USAA)
The United Services Automobile Association (USAA) is a bank and insurance company founded by and for Army officers in 1922 when they were unable to obtain insurance as a result of the perception that they were a high-risk group. Since that time, it has grown to 8.8 million members from all of the military services and branches of government. It offers all banking and brokerage services, credit cards, investment counseling, insurance of all kinds, real estate brokerage, auto buying service, and travel-related services, as well as significant discounts on products and services through retail affiliations and its own mail-order catalog service.

USAA's products and services are offered at significantly better prices than can be found at other retail banks, and because of its conservative investment policies, it was one of the few banks in the United States to emerge from the recent banking crisis unscathed. Further, because of the unique structure of the bank, it pays out dividends annually to its account holders.

The bank has only twenty-two branches nationwide, but it compensates for the lack of banking counters by refunding fees to its members from use of non-USAA ATMs. It also allows members to deposit checks via postage paid envelopes or by submitting photographs of the checks through its online banking system. Members can also conduct all of their transactions, including electronic bill payment, either online at *www.usaa.com* or via its toll-free number, (800) 531-2265.

Shopping

The US Armed Forces run post exchanges (PXs), commissaries (grocery stores), Class VI stores, and fuel stations for the benefit of servicemembers who live at remote bases or don't make much money, or both. The PXs and commissaries sell their merchandise tax-free, often at cost, and are open to all servicemembers and their families. The PXs at larger bases are well stocked and are comparable to midlevel civilian department stores. These PXs often have many other vendors and retail businesses under the same roof, offering everything from flowers to auto servicing. Class VI is the military category for luxury or "personal demand" items, and Class VI stores stock wines, beers, hard liquor, and tobacco products, selling them for a deep discount over civilian retail stores.

The Army and Air Force share their PX, calling it the Army and Air Force Exchange Service (AAFES). The other forces have the Navy Exchange (NEX) and the Coast Guard Exchange (CGX). In reality, however, they are all run by the same company. All can be found on most bases or can be accessed online at shopmyexchange.com, and they generally will ship their products to you for free via FedEx. The military exchanges also have uniform stores so you can order all of your required items online. If you go to the store to purchase them, you will often receive a credit for free tailoring and fitting at the cleaners in the Exchange Mall.

The exchange offers a low-interest credit card called Military Star, which does not report to or check your credit bureau, so it's a good way to get back on your feet if you've had credit troubles. (See *www.shopmyexchange.com/ExchangeCredit.*) In addition, the Star Card puts charges for uniform items in a separate interest-free account, which not only saves you money but also facilitates deduction of uniform purchases at tax time. (While PXs are like department stores, Base Commissaries are grocery stores. The commissary system is contracted separately from AAFES, so it does not accept the Military Star Card.)

Many civilian retail businesses offer military discounts, even though they don't advertise them. For example, Home Depot gives a 25-percent discount if you show your military ID at checkout, and Apple offers 8 percent off computer accessories at its retail stores to shoppers with military IDs. Also, tours, museums, and private clubs often offer free or deeply discounted memberships or access with presentation of an active-duty ID, and national parks give free admission. If you are in uniform in New York City, flashing your ID gets you free access to the subway.

Airport Lounges

The United Services Organization (USO) was founded in 1941 at the request of President Franklin D. Roosevelt to provide morale-building entertainment and services to the US military around the world. It is well remembered for performances by Bob Hope, Marilyn Monroe, and dozens of Hollywood celebrities. Today it continues to provide entertainment to troops the world over, but it also operates soldiers' lounges in major airports around the United States. Servicemembers with IDs can visit the USO lounges to await their planes in comfort. Food, books, lounge chairs, sleeping areas, toiletries, movies, and Internet access are usually available. If you are in uniform and traveling on orders, some commercial airline clubs also will grant you complimentary access to their lounges while you await your plane.

Health and Dental Insurance

Full-time servicemembers are entitled to free medical care at military facilities, as well as at civilian healthcare facilities in the event of emergencies. Additionally, all current Reservists and retired Reserve and full-time servicemembers, their spouses, and children are eligible for TRICARE Health Insurance, which has a variety of plans to fit your specific branch and duty status. The plans are widely accepted by private physicians of your choosing, and they are far less expensive than comparable private plans. As an example, a Reservist who is single and has no children will pay less than $60 a month for full coverage. This benefit alone has been reason enough for some servicemembers to join the military, and you should not take it for granted. TRICARE provides medical prescriptions through Express Scripts, which offers prescription medications at considerable discounts and mails those medications directly to your home. Details on coverage are available at *www.tricare.mil*.

TRICARE Dental is also available for an additional small fee. It covers annual checkups, dental emergencies, and specific procedures. For details, see *www.tricare.mil/dental*.

Education Scholarships

Several educational funding programs are available to servicemembers and their families. The Montgomery and the Post-9/11 GI Bills are the most widely known, but there are a variety of other programs to help you train for a second career or put away money for your children's education. See the Department of Veterans Affairs website, *www.gibill. va.gov/benefits/post_911_gibill/index.html* for information about the programs. These scholarships require that the servicemember has served for a minimum number of years in the full-time or Reserve Army or has completed an overseas deployment for eligibility—in other words, you must be a veteran to be eligible. Note that you do not have to be retired to be a veteran. You can still be an actively drilling Reservist or active-duty soldier and be a veteran. This is an important point to understand, because once you attain veteran status, a clock begins to count down during which time you are able to use your education benefits. If you do not use them within this period, you lose them.

The VA offers so many benefits to veterans that it can become confusing. One of the best ways to ensure that you take advantage of the benefits that you have earned is to speak with a veterans benefits counselor. These individuals are paid as contractors by the VA to help you navigate the system, and thus there is no charge to you. They are located in a variety of settings, often near veterans hospitals, or you can find them through private veterans organizations such as the Veterans of Foreign Wars (VFW). You can also research your benefits online, without the help of a counselor, at *http://benefits.va.gov/benefits*.

If you are not a veteran but are an actively drilling Reservist, state education benefits may be available to you. These benefits vary by state; contact your S1 to learn the specifics. Also see *www.goarmy.com/ reserve/benefits/education.html* if you are in the Reserves or *www. nationalguard.com/life/education-benefits* if you are in the Army National Guard.

ORGANIZATIONS

Military people are good at organizing, so it is not surprising that there are many organizations servicemembers can join. Some are simply social groups, some are advocacy groups, and some provide services. One specifically for medical providers is the Society of Federal Health Professionals, originally the Association of Military Surgeons of the United States (AMSUS), which is the oldest military medical association in the United States, organized in 1891; it currently serves medical professionals in all branches of the armed forces, DoD, and VA.

Most of these organizations can be easily found online by searching for the key words "US Army" or "military" plus your area of interest. For example, searching "US Army" plus "aerospace medicine" brings up the Society for US Army Flight Surgeons (SUSAFS),

Association for Aerospace Medicine (AsMA), and the US Army Aviation Medicine Association (USAAVMA), among others. Other key words to use in your searches are "association," "academy," "organization," and "society."

> ### CORE ORGANIZATIONS
> There are several core organizations that service-members should consider joining.
> - Society of Federal Health Professionals (AMSUS), www.amsus.org
> - Military Officers Association of America (MOAA), www.moaa.org
> - Army Reserve Association (ARA), www.armyreserve.org
> - National Guard Association of the US (NGAUS), www.ngaus.org
> - Veterans of Foreign Wars (VFW), www.vfw.org
> - American Legion, www.legion.org
> - Iraq and Afghanistan Veterans of America (IAVA), www.IAVA.org

Clubs and Hotels
The following clubs and hotels are private organizations unaffiliated with the military, founded to serve current and retired service members.

The Army and Navy Club (ANC), Washington, DC
The Army and Navy Club (ANC) located in Washington, DC was established by veterans of the American Civil War and is the oldest such institution in the United States. Its membership is a "who's who" of American politics, business, and the military. The clubhouse is one block from the White House and houses guestrooms, a sports club, banquet halls, a library, and memorabilia from every campaign from the Civil War to the present. The ANC has reciprocal agreements with many university and private clubs around the world, meaning that members of the ANC are given access as guests to other affiliated clubs (*www.armynavyclub.org*).

The Soldiers', Sailors', Marines', Coast Guard and Airmen's Club, New York City
The Soldiers', Sailors', Marines', Coast Guard and Airmen's Club in New York City was founded in 1919 by General John Pershing and

Mrs. Theodore Roosevelt Jr. to provide accommodations to servicemen returning from service after World War I. Located in a Murray Hill mansion on Lexington Avenue, this private organization provides low-cost subsidized accommodations and club facilities to servicemembers and their families. Whereas the Army and Navy Club is oriented toward wealthy retired officers and provides a classic conservative club atmosphere, this club was founded to provide for younger servicemembers in need of affordable temporary accommodations in the city. It has private and group rooms and is the best deal in the entire city in terms of quality and cost of a hotel room. For details, see *www.ssmaclub.org*.

Marines' Memorial Club and Hotel, San Francisco
This San Francisco hotel was originally built in the 1920s as a women's club but was purchased by a group of Marine veterans during WWII and re-dedicated and re-named to honor fallen Marines in 1946. It functions both as a membership club open to members of all the services and as a hotel open to the public. The building is notable for its central location, large display of military memorabilia, and theater that can seat more than six hundred guests. For more information, visit *www.marine club.com*.

Military Aero Clubs
Military aero clubs are private flying clubs located on military installations. These organizations provide classes and flight time at considerable discounts. There is no central organization for these clubs, so your best bet is to visit the website for the military installation nearest your home and search there for information.

Appendices

Appendix A

Pay and Allowances

The following pay tables present basic military salary based on your pay grade (your enumerated rank) and your years of service. The Monthly Basic Pay table is the reference for officers in the fulltime Active Duty Army. Reserve Component officers must refer to the Reserve Drill Pay table to see their salary for a drill weekend. The tables are updated each financial year and can be accessed at the Defense Finance and Accounting Service website: *www.dfas.mil/ dfas.html.*

The basic salary is often augmented by allowances that compensate for housing expenses, hazardous duty, flight or diving duty, foreign language proficiency, and special skills such as medical, dental, or veterinary degrees. Your paycheck is accompanied by a Leave and Earnings Statement (LES), which enumerates all of the details of your salary. The LES (and annual W-2 forms for taxes) can be accessed at the same DFAS website or directly at *https://mypay.dfas.mil/mypay.aspx.*

For a detailed and clear explanation of military pay, I refer you to *Army Officer's Guide: 52nd Edition*, Appendix A, "Pay and Allowances."

MONTHLY BASIC PAY TABLE (EFFECTIVE JANUARY 1, 2013)

Pay Grade	<2	2	3	4	6	8	10	12	14	16	18	20	22	24	26
Commissioned officers															
O-10[1]												15,913.20	15,990.60	16,323.60	16,902.60
O-9[1]												13,917.60	14,118.60	14,408.10	14,913.30
O-8[1]	9,847.80	10,170.30	10,384.50	10,444.20	10,711.50	11,157.60	11,261.40	11,685.00	11,806.50	12,171.60	12,700.20	13,187.10	13,512.30	13,512.30	13,512.30
O-7[1]	8,182.50	8,562.90	8,738.70	8,878.50	9,131.70	9,381.90	9,671.40	9,959.40	10,248.60	11,157.60	11,924.70	11,924.70	11,924.70	11,924.70	11,985.60
O-6[2]	6,064.80	6,663.00	7,100.10	7,100.10	7,127.10	7,432.80	7,473.00	7,473.00	7,897.80	8,648.70	9,089.40	9,529.80	9,780.60	10,034.40	10,526.70
O-5	5,055.90	5,695.50	6,089.70	6,164.10	6,410.10	6,557.10	6,880.80	7,118.40	7,425.30	7,895.10	8,118.00	8,338.80	8,589.90	8,589.90	8,589.90
O-4	4,362.30	5,049.90	5,386.80	5,461.80	5,774.70	6,109.80	6,527.70	6,852.90	7,078.80	7,208.70	7,283.70	7,283.70	7,283.70	7,283.70	7,283.70
O-3	3,835.50	4,347.90	4,692.90	5,116.50	5,361.60	5,630.70	5,804.70	6,090.60	6,240.00	6,240.00	6,240.00	6,240.00	6,240.00	6,240.00	6,240.00
O-2	3,314.10	3,774.30	4,347.00	4,493.70	4,586.40	4,586.40	4,586.40	4,586.40	4,586.40	4,586.40	4,586.40	4,586.40	4,586.40	4,586.40	4,586.40
O-1	2,876.40	2,994.00	3,619.20	3,619.20	3,619.20	3,619.20	3,619.20	3,619.20	3,619.20	3,619.20	3,619.20	3,619.20	3,619.20	3,619.20	3,619.20
Commissioned officers with over 4 years active duty service as an enlisted member or warrant officer															
O-3[3]				5,116.50	5,361.60	5,630.70	5,804.70	6,090.60	6,332.10	6,470.70	6,659.40	6,659.40	6,659.40	6,659.40	6,659.40
O-2[3]				4,493.70	4,586.40	4,732.50	4,978.80	5,169.30	5,311.20	5,311.20	5,311.20	5,311.20	5,311.20	5,311.20	5,311.20
O-1[3]				3,619.20	3,864.60	4,007.70	4,153.80	4,297.20	4,493.70	4,493.70	4,493.70	4,493.70	4,493.70	4,493.70	4,493.70
Warrant officers															
W-5								5,439.60	5,713.50	5,974.20	6,187.50	7,047.90	7,405.50	7,671.60	7,966.50
W-4	3,963.90	4,263.90	4,386.00	4,506.60	4,713.90	4,919.10	5,126.70	5,439.60	5,713.50	5,974.20	6,187.50	6,395.40	6,701.10	6,952.20	7,238.70
W-3	3,619.50	3,770.40	3,925.20	3,975.90	4,138.20	4,457.10	4,789.20	4,945.50	5,126.40	5,313.00	5,648.10	5,874.30	6,009.90	6,153.90	6,349.50
W-2	3,202.80	3,505.80	3,599.40	3,663.30	3,871.20	4,194.00	4,353.90	4,511.40	4,704.00	4,854.30	4,990.80	5,153.70	5,261.10	5,346.30	5,346.30
W-1	2,811.60	3,114.00	3,195.30	3,367.50	3,570.90	3,870.60	4,010.40	4,205.70	4,398.30	4,549.80	4,689.00	4,858.20	4,858.20	4,858.20	4,858.20
Enlisted members															
E-9[4]							4,788.90	4,897.50	5,034.30	5,194.80	5,357.40	5,617.50	5,837.10	6,068.70	6,422.70
E-8						3,920.10	4,093.50	4,200.90	4,329.60	4,469.10	4,720.50	4,847.70	5,064.60	5,184.90	5,481.00
E-7	2,725.20	2,974.50	3,088.20	3,239.10	3,357.00	3,559.20	3,673.20	3,875.70	4,043.70	4,158.60	4,281.00	4,328.40	4,487.40	4,572.90	4,897.80
E-6	2,357.10	2,593.80	2,708.10	2,819.40	2,935.50	3,196.50	3,298.50	3,495.30	3,555.60	3,599.70	3,650.70	3,650.70	3,650.70	3,650.70	3,650.70
E-5	2,159.40	2,304.30	2,415.90	2,529.90	2,707.50	2,893.50	3,045.60	3,064.20	3,064.20	3,064.20	3,064.20	3,064.20	3,064.20	3,064.20	3,064.20
E-4	1,979.70	2,081.10	2,193.90	2,304.90	2,403.30	2,403.30	2,403.30	2,403.30	2,403.30	2,403.30	2,403.30	2,403.30	2,403.30	2,403.30	2,403.30
E-3	1,787.40	1,899.90	2,014.80	2,014.80	2,014.80	2,014.80	2,014.80	2,014.80	2,014.80	2,014.80	2,014.80	2,014.80	2,014.80	2,014.80	2,014.80
E-2	1,699.80	1,699.80	1,699.80	1,699.80	1,699.80	1,699.80	1,699.80	1,699.80	1,699.80	1,699.80	1,699.80	1,699.80	1,699.80	1,699.80	1,699.80
E-1[5]	1,516.20														

NOTES:

1. Basic pay for an O-7 to O-10 is limited by Level II of the Executive Schedule which is $14,975.10. Basic pay for O-6 and below is limited by Level V of the Executive Schedule which is $12,141.60.
2. While serving as Chairman, Joint Chief of Staff/Vice Chairman, Joint Chief of Staff, Chief of Navy Operations, Commandant of the Marine Corps, Army/Air Force Chief of Staff, Commander of a unified or specified combatant command, basic pay is $20,937.90. (See note 1 above).
3. Applicable to O-1 to O-3 with at least 4 years and 1 day of active duty or more than 1460 points as a warrant and/or enlisted member. See Department of Defense Financial Management Regulations for more detailed explanation on who is eligible for this special basic pay rate.
4. For the Master Chief Petty Officer of the Navy, Chief Master Sergeant of the AF, Sergeant Major of the Army or Marine Corps or Senior Enlisted Advisor of the JCS, basic pay is $7,738.80. Combat Zone Tax Exclusion for O-1 and above is based on this basic pay rate plus Hostile Fire Pay/Imminent Danger Pay which is $225.00.
5. Applicable to E-1 with 4 months or more of active duty. Basic pay for an E-1 with less than 4 months of active duty is $1,402.20.
6. Basic pay rate for Academy Cadets/Midshipmen and ROTC members/applicants is $1,006.80.

RESERVE DRILL PAY (FOUR DRILL PERIODS)
(EFFECTIVE 1 JANUARY 2013)

Years of Service

Grade	<2	2	3	4	6	8	10	12	14	16	18	20	22	24	26
Commissioned officers															
O-7	8,182.50	8,562.90	8,738.70	8,878.50	9,131.70	9,381.90	9,671.10	9,959.40	10,248.60	11,157.60	11,924.70	11,924.70	11,924.70	11,924.70	11,985.60
O-6	6,064.80	6,663.00	7,100.10	7,100.10	7,127.10	7,432.80	7,473.00	7,473.00	7,897.80	8,648.70	9,089.40	9,529.80	9,780.60	10,034.40	10,526.70
O-5	5,055.90	5,695.50	6,089.70	6,164.10	6,410.10	6,557.10	6,880.80	7,118.40	7,425.30	7,895.10	8,118.00	8,338.80	8,589.90	8,589.90	8,589.90
O-4	4,362.30	5,049.90	5,386.80	5,461.80	5,774.70	6,109.80	6,527.70	6,852.90	7,078.80	7,208.70	7,283.70	7,283.70	7,283.70	7,283.70	7,283.70
O-3	3,835.50	4,347.90	4,692.90	5,116.50	5,361.60	5,630.70	5,804.70	6,090.60	6,240.00	6,240.00	6,240.00	6,240.00	6,240.00	6,240.00	6,240.00
O-2	3,314.10	3,774.30	4,347.00	4,493.70	4,586.40	4,586.40	4,586.40	4,586.40	4,586.40	4,586.40	4,586.40	4,586.40	4,586.40	4,586.40	4,586.40
O-1	2,876.40	2,994.00	3,619.20	3,619.20	3,619.20	3,619.20	3,619.20	3,619.20	3,619.20	3,619.20	3,619.20	3,619.20	3,619.20	3,619.20	3,619.20
Commissioned officers with over 4 years active duty service as an enlisted member or warrant officer															
O-3E				5,116.50	5,361.60	5,630.70	5,804.70	6,090.60	6,332.10	6,470.70	6,659.40	6,659.40	6,659.40	6,659.40	6,659.40
O-2E				4,493.70	4,586.40	4,732.50	4,978.80	5,169.30	5,311.20	5,311.20	5,311.20	5,311.20	5,311.20	5,311.20	5,311.20
O-1E				3,619.20	3,864.60	4,007.70	4,153.80	4,297.20	4,493.70	4,493.70	4,493.70	4,493.70	4,493.70	4,493.70	4,493.70
Warrant officers															
W-5												7,047.90	7,405.50	7,671.60	7,966.50
W-4	3,963.90	4,263.90	4,386.00	4,506.60	4,713.90	4,919.10	5,126.70	5,439.60	5,713.50	5,974.20	6,187.50	6,395.40	6,701.10	6,952.20	7,238.70
W-3	3,619.50	3,770.40	3,925.20	3,975.90	4,138.20	4,457.10	4,789.20	4,945.50	5,126.40	5,313.00	5,648.10	5,874.30	6,009.90	6,153.90	6,349.50
W-2	3,202.80	3,505.80	3,599.40	3,663.30	3,871.20	4,194.00	4,353.90	4,511.40	4,704.00	4,854.30	4,990.80	5,153.70	5,261.10	5,346.30	5,346.30
W-1	2,811.60	3,114.00	3,195.30	3,367.50	3,570.90	3,870.60	4,010.40	4,205.70	4,398.30	4,549.80	4,689.00	4,858.20	4,858.20	4,858.20	4,858.20
Enlisted members															
E-9							4,788.90	4,897.50	5,054.30	5,194.80	5,357.40	5,617.50	5,837.10	6,068.70	6,422.70
E-8						3,920.10	4,093.50	4,200.90	4,329.60	4,469.10	4,720.50	4,847.70	5,064.60	5,184.90	5,481.00
E-7	2,725.20	2,974.50	3,088.20	3,239.10	3,357.00	3,559.20	3,673.20	3,875.70	4,003.70	4,158.60	4,281.00	4,328.40	4,487.40	4,572.90	4,897.80
E-6	2,357.10	2,593.80	2,708.10	2,819.40	2,935.50	3,196.50	3,298.50	3,495.30	3,555.60	3,599.70	3,650.70	3,650.70	3,650.70	3,650.70	3,650.70
E-5	2,159.40	2,304.30	2,415.90	2,529.90	2,707.50	2,893.50	3,045.60	3,064.20	3,064.20	3,064.20	3,064.20	3,064.20	3,064.20	3,064.20	3,064.20
E-4	1,979.70	2,081.10	2,193.90	2,304.90	2,403.30	2,403.30	2,403.30	2,403.30	2,403.30	2,403.30	2,403.30	2,403.30	2,403.30	2,403.30	2,403.30
E-3	1,787.40	1,899.90	2,014.80	2,014.80	2,014.80	2,014.80	2,014.80	2,014.80	2,014.80	2,014.80	2,014.80	2,014.80	2,014.80	2,014.80	2,014.80
E-2	1,699.80	1,699.80	1,699.80	1,699.80	1,699.80	1,699.80	1,699.80	1,699.80	1,699.80	1,699.80	1,699.80	1,699.80	1,699.80	1,699.80	1,699.80
E-1 >4 mos	1,516.20														
E-1 <4 mos	1,402.20														

Appendix B

Travel and Recreation

The military life is one of dedication and sacrifice, so it is fitting that the military offers many opportunities for travel and recreation for active and retired servicemembers and their families.

MORALE, WELFARE, AND RECREATION (MWR)

Morale, welfare, and recreation (MWR) refers to military-sponsored off-time activities. Most bases have MWR centers, though the services they offer depend on the population and nature of the base. Larger bases have gyms, pools, recreational vehicles, bicycles, boats, movie theaters, bowling alleys, water activities on beaches, lakes and rivers, and fitness and activities classes, and can also arrange tours of the local area.

SPACE-AVAILABLE, OR SPACE-A

The military allows its full-time, Reserve, and retired members to stay in military lodging and travel on military aircraft when space is available. Active-duty, Reserve Component, and retired servicemembers are permitted to travel free of charge as passengers on military aircraft that are carrying out nontactical missions.

If you are active-duty or Reserve Component and wish to travel space-available, or Space-A, you must have DD Form 1853, Verification of Reserve Status for Travel Eligibility, signed by an NCO or commander within six months of your trip. This form notifies the personnel at the air terminal that you are authorized to travel on a military aircraft. If you are entering a military base or recreation area, you do not need Form 1853 but you do need to present your military ID or retired servicemember ID.

All flights depart from PAX terminals, many of which resemble commercial terminals (but considerably less crowded) on military bases. The seating is on a Space-A basis, meaning that if there is room left over on the plane after cargo and mission-bound personnel have been loaded, passenger seats will be made available. Military aircraft that move cargo and personnel into and out of the theater of operations notify the PAX terminal staff of extra seats that they have available. The PAX terminal staff post available flights on a video monitor, along with the available seats. You can also call in for a telephone recording that lists the daily departures and arrivals at each terminal with seats available, updated daily. The available seats are prioritized and then given out on a first-come, first-served basis (see DoD 4515.13-R, Air Transportation Eligibility).

To get a Space-A seat, military personnel and authorized contractors present themselves to the PAX dispatch desk and request a seat on a flight. Those who are granted either a seat or a place on the waiting list are informed of the "show-time." Individuals hoping to travel on the flight must return to the PAX terminal at "show-time," at which point they will be notified if the flight is still scheduled and if they have seats on that flight. If you are given a seat, you present your CAC and DD Form 1853 to the dispatch desk, you are manifested on the flight, and you are given a roll-call time, at which point you must be present with all of your gear, ready to travel. If not given a seat, you need to repeat the process, returning to the PAX terminal every few hours to check the monitors for available flights. Alternatively, it is now possible—and even encouraged—to sign up for flights online at *www.takeahop.com*, rather than simply show up at the PAX terminal in hopes of getting a seat.

Seating on these planes can range from commercial-type seats to cargo net seating, and you may be flying on a small passenger plane, large commercial passenger plane, aerial refueler, or large cargo aircraft. The cargo aircraft are pressurized but are very noisy and often quite cold, so earplugs, extra layers, and a seat cushion are recommended. Inexpensive cold box lunches are sometimes available for sale at the ticket counter and will be delivered to you on the aircraft.

MILITARY LODGING
Each of the services runs inns or lodges on military bases across the country that cater to visiting military families and active and retired personnel. Some of these lodges are located in spectacular locations, including Honolulu; Washington, DC; New York City; Cape Cod, Massachusetts; and San Juan, Puerto Rico. The lodgings are comparable to those at civilian motels but are considerably cheaper. For details, see *www.dodlodging.net*.

ARMED FORCES RECREATION CENTERS (AFRCS)

Armed Forces Recreation Centers (AFRCs) are resorts located around the world that cater specifically to the military and their families. These resorts are quite popular, for obvious reasons, so reservations far in advance are recommended. AFRC room rates are affordable and based on rank, pay grade, duty status, and room size and location.

> Shades of Green, Walt Disney World Resort, Florida, www.shadesofgreen.org
> Edelweiss Lodge and Resort, Germany, www.edelweisslodgeandresort.com
> Hale Koa Hotel, Hawaii, www.halekoa.com
> Dragon Hill Lodge, Korea, www.dragonhilllodge.com
> The New Sanno Hotel, Tokyo, Japan, www.thenewsanno.com

TRAVEL RESOURCES FOR MILITARY PERSONNEL

The following are some travel and vacation resources for military personnel:

> US Army MWR, www.armymwr.com/travel
> Government and Armed Forces Travel Cooperative, www.govarm.com
> Armed Forces Vacation Club, www.afvclub.com
> Military Living, www.militaryliving.com
> John D's Military Space-Available Travel Pages, www.spacea.net
> Dirk Pepperd's Space-A Message Board, www.pepperd.com/vb/usercp.php

Appendix C

Uniforms and Appearance

Most Army officers still remember the first time they put on their uniforms. More than just a suit of clothes you hang on your frame, the uniform physically changes you. It transforms your body, improving your posture, straightening your back, and lengthening your stride. People behave differently toward you, because your uniform transforms you into a man or woman who is a symbol of our military and its history. Your behavior also changes, because you are aware that you are being watched and are being judged as a military officer. You may suddenly find yourself thinking twice about crossing the street against a light, walking down the street while eating, or having another drink. The uniform is also a powerful recruitment tool, because when worn properly, it makes you look powerful and charismatic, and people want to be with you. The Marines have known this for years and take pains to make sure their young recruits look sharp when they return from basic training, knowing that the newly minted Marines will make their moms, girlfriends, and boyfriends proud and friends jealous, thus generating new recruits.

The Army has recently rediscovered the value of a sharp uniform and has reintroduced the traditional Dress Blue Uniform. The Dress Blue, now known as the Class A and Class B Army Service Uniform (ASU) is a variation of the uniform that was worn by the Union Army during the Civil War period, and it looks great. Officers wear a dark blue coat and light "cavalry blue" pants, with gold buttons, gold stripes on their legs, and gold-rimmed shoulder boards displaying their rank. It is new enough that the general public often mistakes Army officers for Marine officers—which we outwardly hate but inwardly like.

When you are sworn in as an officer, you receive along with your first paycheck a onetime clothing allowance with which you are to purchase the basic uniform items. The amount varies, but it is generally around $300. Upon commissioning, Army Reserve officers are also given a uniform allowance of a few hundred dollars. The allowance is not enough money to purchase everything, but it makes a dent in the overall bill. Uniform items throughout your career are not taxed if purchased at a military uniform store, and you can deduct the total cost from your income taxes.

UNIFORMS AND ACCESSORIES

You are required to own and maintain the Class A and B Army Service Uniforms (ASU), the Army Combat Uniform (ACU), and the Physical Training Uniform (PTU). Many options and accessories are available, but at the beginning of your career, it is advisable to concentrate on acquiring the basic uniforms and learning to wear them correctly. If you subsequently have an interest in broadening your wardrobe, consult AR 670-1, Wear and Appearance of the Army Uniform.

The current secretary of the Army has directed his staff to begin wearing the Class A and B as their day-to-day uniforms at the Pentagon. It is the commander's prerogative to determine the uniform for his troops. Most Reserve and Guard Army units continue to wear the ACU as their regular uniform.

You are required to purchase the following:

- Class A Uniform: blue coat with rank, US, AMEDD, and specialty insignia and nameplate; light blue slacks with gold stripe; black elastic uniform belt with gold buckle; long-sleeved white uniform shirt with rank and nameplate; long black tie; black patent leather uniform shoes; black socks; and either a brim hat with gold officer eagle or a beret with rank

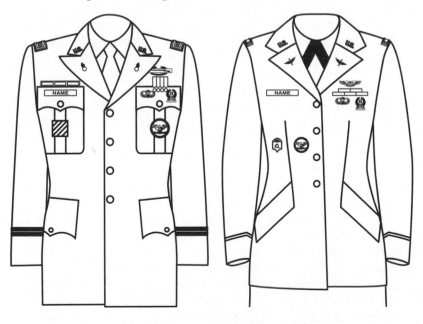

Men's and Women's Blue Army Service Uniform Coat

- Class B Uniform: light blue slacks with gold stripe and belt (these are the same as in the Class A Uniform, so you don't have to buy two pairs); short-sleeved white shirt with rank and name-plate; shoes; and a hat (both the latter are the same as in the Class A; no tie required

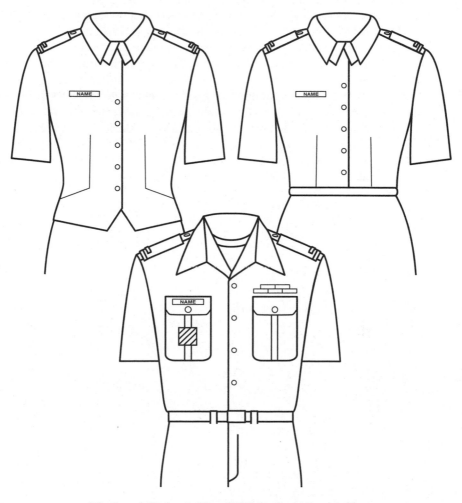

Men's and Women's Class B White short-sleeved shirt

- Army Combat Uniform (ACU): camouflage blouse with rank, unit (supplied by your unit if not available at the uniform store), and American flag patches; matching pants; tan web belt; three light brown T-shirts; brown suede combat boots; brown or green tube socks; and a field cap with sew-on or pin-on rank
- Physical Training Uniform (PTU): long-sleeved gray Army T-shirt; short-sleeved Army T-shirt; black Army shorts; gray Army jacket; black pants; reflective belt; running shoes (any brand); white socks that cover the ankles; and a green fleece winter hat
- Optional items: black short windbreaker with rank to wear with Class B; long black trench coat with rank to wear over Class A or B (men are not permitted to carry umbrellas for themselves while in uniform); V-neck pullover or cardigan sweater with rank to be worn with the Class B uniform; and an AMEDD crest and nameplate.

At a bare minimum, get the required items above, have them fitted as necessary, and look professional when you first show up to your unit

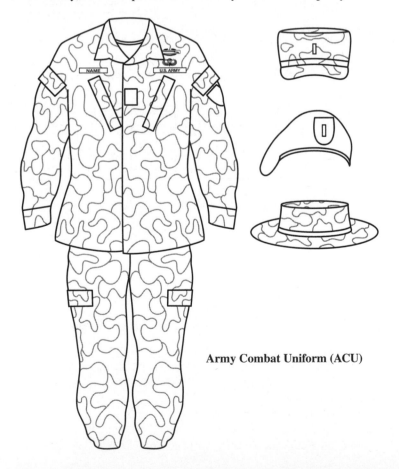

Army Combat Uniform (ACU)

and present yourself to your commander. Your first impression in uniform as an officer is extremely important and sets the tone for your job. If you show up looking sloppy, your troops will get the message that you are not informed and don't pay attention to details. It will undermine their respect for you and degrade their work.

The details of the US Army uniforms are covered in AR 670-1, which explains the items in each uniform. It is available for free online, and it is a good idea to download this and thumb through it. You can also find books that explain proper wear and appearance. You may be surprised at the variety of uniforms available, from hospital whites to judges' robes. You may wish to obtain the formal blue or white uniforms, which you can wear instead of a tuxedo on formal social occasions.

The rest of the equipment assigned to you as a soldier and officer is referred to as TA-50, for Table of Allowances. These items used to be called "General Issue," hence the nickname GIs for soldiers that arose during World War II. When you are assigned to your unit, the duty sergeant will assign you your TA-50 from the Central Issuing Facility (CIF). Although you take possession of this equipment and sign a hand receipt for it, it remains the property of the US Army. You are expected to use and return it when it is worn out or you retire. If any items are missing, you must pay for them. If you are assigned to a fixed facility that never goes out to the field, you can decline the TA-50 until you need it. You will need certain items annually, however. For example, you will go to the range to fire a weapon once or twice a year, for which you will need a helmet, safety glasses, and vest. Your duty sergeant will guide you regarding equipment.

If you are deployed with your unit, it will issue all your gear. If you are deployed as an individual, you will report to a deployment center where you will be issued gear—either a complete kit or items to supplement those you were instructed to bring.

Each item of Army equipment and clothing has instructions attached. Read and follow them. The winter gear, for example, is extremely well designed and expensive. It is very effective but must be worn and cleaned properly. As a medical officer, it is part of your job to understand this and instruct your medics and troops on how to properly use the winter gear to prevent cold injuries. You are permitted to wear your issued gear when not on duty, but you must remove rank and unit identification.

DOG TAGS

ID tags, commonly called dog tags, are often made at the home unit, although you can have them made at your own expense at any time. Dog tags are considered to be part of your uniform and should be worn whenever you are on duty, especially if you are flying. Each soldier is issued two of them so that if he or she is killed, one can stay on the body while the other is collected by the medic to be delivered to the person responsible for tracking soldiers killed in action (KIAs) and initiating the casualty reporting system.

WHERE AND HOW TO PURCHASE UNIFORMS

Enlisted troops receive their uniforms when they attend basic training. Officers must procure their own and are expected to wear them properly immediately upon reporting for duty. There are several options for purchasing the uniform. The Army and Air Force Exchange Service (AAFES) Uniform Centers carry all of the required uniform items. You can visit the stores and avail yourself of the assistance offered by the staff, or you can order your uniforms through the AAFES website, *www.shopmyexchange.com*, or one of various retailers. Marlow White (*www.marlowwhite.com*) is one of the most well-known, high-quality custom uniform companies.

Although it may be tempting to do your shopping online, it is recommended that you go in person to a military clothing store, preferably with someone who is already in the service to guide you (your recruiter may do this for you), so that you can try on the items and have them fitted. Another advantage to going to the store is that the staff will walk you through what you need and make sure everything is assembled correctly.

AAFES will give you a certificate for free tailoring after you purchase your uniform, but wherever you purchase your uniform, be sure to have it fitted. A poorly fitting uniform looks terrible and makes you appear unprofessional. Uniform pants must be exactly the right length and must not bunch up in the leg; just because they button around your waist does not mean they fit properly. Uniform jackets must hang straight and sheath your torso, not drown it. Military tailors will also make sure that your insignia are correct and put on in the right places.

SPECIAL UNIFORMS

Medical providers may also be issued or required to buy special uniforms if they receive assignments or training that require special gear. For example, flight surgeons are issued flame-retardant flight suits. Hospital personnel in fixed facilities may be issued and authorized to wear hospital whites, scrubs, and lab coats.

Be aware that although the hospital commander has the authority to determine the uniform policy within the medical facility, that authority ends when medical personnel step out of the facility. In other words, the commander may permit the Emergency Department staff to remove their blouses and work in T-shirts or to walk the hospital grounds without their weapons. Once off the hospital grounds, base policy prevails, and you must wear the uniform and additional items as proscribed by the base commander.

Appendix D

Professional References and Reading Guide

If you are deploying on a mission with a unit, funds may be available for you to purchase medical references for your use. The supply NCO has a list of items that may be ordered for deployment, and if it includes medical reference books, no extra funds will be necessary. Deploying units often are given discretionary funds, so if there is a reference that you think is crucial to the mission, request the funds from your commander or executive officer (XO). If you are deploying as an individual and would like to purchase references and attend training before deployment, contact your State Surgeon's Office and ask for assistance.

It is strongly recommended that you consider the environment in which you will be practicing before ordering books. If you are deploying as an individual, you will be carrying your own bags, which will already be overstuffed and heavy. In this case, electronic books on your computer, reading tablet, or USB flash drive would be a superior choice. If, however, you are deploying to a location that does not have reliable power, then books (preferably paperback) are a better choice. If you are deploying with an entire unit that is shipping its gear to its duty station, then putting some books in the shipping containers will not be a problem.

The following list of official references is a compilation of the publications that are the most relevant for the newly commissioned medical officer; it does not contain every publication produced for and by AMEDD or related agencies. Most of these publications, along with a more complete list of all nonclassified Army publications, can be found in PDF format at *http://armypubs.army.mil/index.html*. The posters and technical guides are available at *www.usaphcapps.amedd.army.mil*. It is highly recommended that you download all of the regulations onto a computer, tablet, or smartphone for future reference.

Those publications listed below that are not available at the Army publications website have their sources listed with them.

ARMY REGULATIONS
AR 40-13, Radiological Advisory Medical Teams
AR 40-21, Medical Aspects of Army Aircraft Accident Investigation
AR 40-3, Medical, Dental, and Veterinary Care
AR 40-400, Patient Administration
AR 40-5, Preventive Medicine
AR 40-501, Standards of Medical Fitness
AR 40-562, Immunizations and Chemoprophylaxis
AR 40-66, Medical Record Administration and Health Care Documentation
AR 40-8, Temporary Flying Restrictions Due to Exogenous Factors Affecting Aircrew Efficiency
AR 600-60, Physical Performance Evaluation System
AR 635-40, Physical Evaluation for Retention, Retirement, or Separation

ARMY DIRECTIVE
2012-20, Physical Fitness and Height and Weight Requirements for Professional Military Education

ARMY TECHNICAL PUBLICATION
ATP 4-15.13, Casualty Evacuation

ARMY TACTICS, TECHNIQUES, AND PROCEDURES
ATTP 4-02, Army Health System

FIELD MANUALS
FM 21-10, Field Hygiene and Sanitation
FM 4-02.12, Army Health System Command and Control Organizations
FM 4-02.18, Veterinary Service: Tactics, Techniques, and Procedures
FM 4-02.2, Medical Evacuation
FM 4-02.25, Employment of Forward Surgical Teams: Tactics, Techniques, and Procedures
FM 4-02.283, Treatment of Nuclear and Radiological Casualties
FM 4-02.43, Force Health Protection Support for Army Special Operations Forces

FM 4-02.46, Medical Support of Detainee Operations
FM 4-02.51, Combat and Operation Stress Control
FM 4-02.6 (8-10-1), The Medical Company: Tactics, Techniques, and Procedures
FM 4-02.7, Preventive Medicine Services
FM 4-2.1, Army Medical Logistics
FM 4-2.10, Theater Hospitalization
FM 8-10, Health Service Support in a Theater of Operations
FM 8-10-5, Brigade and Division Surgeons' Handbook: Tactics, Techniques, and Procedures
FM 8-10-6, Medical Evacuation in a Theater of Operations
FM 8-10-19, Dental Service Support in a Theater of Operations
FM 8-284, Treatment of Biological Warfare Agent Casualties
FM 8-40, Management of Skin Diseases in the Tropics
FM 8-42, Medical Operations in Low Intensity Conflict
FM 8-51, Combat Stress Control in a Theater of Operations

NATIONAL GUARD REGULATIONS
NGR 600-200, Enlisted Personnel Management

MEDICAL COMMAND REGULATIONS
MEDCOM Reg 40-28, U.S. Army Veterinary Command Policies and Procedures
MEDCOM Reg 40-36, Medical Facility Management of Sexual Assault
MEDCOM Reg 40-38, Command Directed Mental Health Evaluations
MEDCOM Reg 40-51, Army Substance Abuse Program

PAMPHLETS
PAM 40-501, Hearing Conservation Program
PAM 40-506, The Army Vision Conservation and Readiness Program

TECHNICAL BULLETINS
TB MED 287, Pseudofolliculitis of the Beard
TB MED 289, Aeromedical Evacuation: A Guide for Healthcare Providers
TB MED 505, Altitude Acclimatization and Illness Management
TB MED 507, Heat Stress Control and Heat Casualty Management
TB MED 508, Prevention and Management of Cold Weather Injuries

TRAINING MANUAL
> TM 8-227-12, Armed Services Blood Program Joint Blood Program Handbook

POSTERS
> USACHPPM Poster CP-025-0810, Arachnids of Afghanistan
> USACHPPM Poster CP-033-0811, Work/Rest Water Consumption Table

TECHNICAL GUIDES
> TG 273, Diagnosis and Treatment of Diseases of Tactical Importance to CENTCOM
> TG 336, Malaria Field Guide
> TG 244, The Medical CBRN (Chemical, Biological, Radiation, Nuclear) Battlebook, ISBN-13 9781616082789, Special Operations Forces Medical Handbook

CDS
> NAVMEDPUB 5139, Health Care in Military Settings
> NCMI MEDIC CD, Medical Intelligence Disease Intelligence and Countermeasures

NEWSLETTERS FOR PROFESSIONAL DEVELOPMENT
> Army, www.armymedicine.army.mil/news/mercury/mercury.cfm
> Navy, www.med.navy.mil/sites/navmedmpte/cme

AMEDD VIRTUAL LIBRARY
The AMEDD Virtual Library is a website that gives Army Medical officers free access to hundreds of medical and nursing textbooks, journals, and databases, including UpToDate, Cochrane, and PubMed. To prevent unauthorized use, you can access it only by first accessing your AKO account and then going to *https://medlinet.amedd.army.mil* on a separate page. The website also provides portals to other online book sources. The Virtual Library is a practical alternative to carrying books with you on deployment, but make sure you will have reliable computer access before deciding to rely on it. The Navy has a similar website, *www.med.navy.mil/sites/nmcp/library/pages/telelibrary.aspx*.

BORDEN INSTITUTE MILITARY MEDICINE TEXTBOOKS
The Borden Institute, at Walter Reed Army Medical Center in Washington, DC, publishes textbooks that are authoritative works covering a

whole range of medical specialties from a military perspective. The books are available for free to medical officers as PDF downloads and also as printed books, many in beautiful leatherbound volumes. Borden also publishes military history and specialty titles, which have included *War Surgery in Iraq and Afghanistan: A Series of Cases, 2003–2007*, and *Pediatric Surgery and Medicine in Hostile Environments*. Visit *www.Bordeninstitute.army.mil*.

MILITARY MEDICAL WEBSITES

Public Health Command, preventive health, http://phc.amedd.army.mil

Air Force/Interservice Medical Reference, www.au.af.mil/au/awc/awcgate/awc-medi.htm

Army Insect Vector Information, www.afpmb.org

Air Force Patient Movement Tracker, www.trac2es.transcom.mil

TRICARE Mail Order Pharmacy, www.express-scripts.com/TRICARE

Theater Medical Data Store (TMDS), access to military medical records, https://tmds.tmip.osd.mil

Army Course Catalog, www.atrrs.army.mil/atrrscc

Defense Language Institute Foreign Language Center (DLIFLC), country culture orientation guides and language instruction, www.dliflc.edu/products.html

Army Medical Specialist Corps Deployment Readiness Handbook, www.scribd.com/doc/24591061/Army-Medical-Specialist-Corps-Deployment-Readiness-Handbook-December-1999

Servicemembers Group Life Insurance (SGLI), benefits.va.gov/insurance/sgli.asp

Thrift Savings Plan (TSP), www.tsp.gov/index.shtml

Suggestions to the Command Sergeant Major of the Army, armysuggestions.army.mil

LESSONS LEARNED

Army Lessons Learned, http://usacac.army.mil/cac2/call/index.asp

Army Medical Lessons Learned, http://lessonslearned.amedd.army.mil

Navy Medical Lessons Learned, www.med.navy.mil/bumed/pages/navymedicinelessonslearned.aspx

Air Force Medical Lessons Learned, http://www.au.af.mil/au/awc/awcgate/awc-lesn.htm

MEDICAL INTELLIGENCE RESOURCES
Armed Forces Medical Intelligence Center (AFMIC)
  Fort Detrick, MD
  COMM 301-663-9154 AV 343-7154

Naval Environmental Preventive Medicine Units (NEPMU)
  NEPMU 2 Norfolk, VA
  COM 804-444-7671 AV 654-7671
  NEPMU 5 San Diego, CA
  COMM 619-556-7070
  NEPMU 6 Pearl Harbor, HI
  COMM 808-471-9505 AV 471-9505
  NEPMU 7 Naples, Italy
  COMM 011-39-81-724-4468 ext 4468

Walter Reed Army Institute of Research (WRAIR)
  Washington, DC
  COMM 202-576-3517/3553 AV 291-3517/3553

US Army Special Operations Command
  Office of the Command Surgeon
  Attn: Medical Intelligence Section
  Fort Bragg, NC 28307
  COMM 910-432-5883/9829
  FAX 910-432-4292

Centers for Disease Control
  www.cdc.gov/travel

CIA Factbook
  www.cia.gov/library/publications/the-world-factbook/geos/xx.html

World Health Organization
  www.who.int/ith/en

International Society for Infectious Disease, or Promed
  www.promedmail.org

EMAIL ADDRESSES FOR MEDICAL CONSULTATIONS
  Cardiology   cards.consult@us.army.mil
  Dermatology   derm.consult@us.army.mil
  Burn trauma   burntrauma.consult@us.army.mil

Infectious diseases	id.consult@us.army.mil
Infection control	infect.cntrl.consult@us.army.mil
Internal medicine	im.consult@us.army.mil
Laboratory services	microbiology.consult@us.army.mil
Nephrology	nephrology.consult@us.army.mil
Neurology	neuron.consult@us.army.mil
Ophthalmology and optometry	eye.consult@us.army.mil
Orthopedics and podiatry	ortho.consult@us.army.mil
Pediatrics intensive care	picu.consult@us.army. mil
Preventive medicine	pmom.consult@us.army.mil
Rheumatology	rheum.consult@us.army.mil
Sleep medicine	sleep.e.consult@us.army.mil
Traumatic brain injury	tbi.consult@us.army.mil
Toxicology	toxicology.consult@us.army.mil
Urology	urology.consult@us.army.mil

Appendix E

Glossary

ACRONYMS AND ABBREVIATIONS

AAFES	Army and Air Force Exchange Service
ACU	Army Combat Uniform
ADT	active-duty training
AMEDD	Army Medical Department
AO	area of operations
AOC	area of concentration
APC	Army personnel carrier
APFT	Army Physical Fitness Test
AR	Army Regulation
ARNG	Army National Guard
ASMC	area support medical company
ASU	Army Service Uniform
AWOL	absent without leave
BAH	basic allowance for housing
BAS	battalion aid station; basic allowance for subsistence
BCT	brigade combat team
BOG	Boots on Ground (time in combat)
BOQ	bachelor officers' quarters
CAB	Combat Action Badge
CAC	common access card; Combined Arms Center
CIB	Combat Infantryman Badge
CID	Criminal Investigation Division
CLASS I	food, comfort items
CLASS II	individual equipment
CLASS III	fuel, lubricants
CLASS IV	construction materials
CLASS V	ammunition, ordnance
CLASS VI	alcohol, personal items
CLASS VII	vehicles
CLASS VIII	medical materiel

CLASS IX	repair, maintenance
CLASS X	non-military materiel
COL	colonel
COLA	cost of living allowance
CONUS	continental United States
CPL	corporal
CPT	captain
CSH	combat support hospital
CSM	command sergeant major
CTA	Common Table of Allowances
DA	Department of the Army
DEERS	Defense Enrollment Eligibility Reporting System
DENCOM	Dental Command
DFAC	dining facility
DoD or DD	Department of Defense (DD is used for forms)
DUI	distinctive uniform (or unit) insignia
EFMB	Expert Field Medical Badge
EIB	Expert Infantry Badge
EOD	explosive ordnance disposal
FHA	Federal Housing Authority
FM	Field Manual
FSMC	forward support medical company
FST	forward surgical team; fire support team
FTX	field training exercise
GEN	general
GSA	General Services Administration
GTA	graphical training aid
HHC	Headquarters and Headquarters Company
HOR	Home of Record
HQ	headquarters
IB	infantry brigade
ICTB	Interfacility Credentials Transfer Brief
IED	improvised explosive device
IG	inspector general
INF	infantry
JAG	judge advocate general
JRTC	Joint Readiness Training Center
KP	kitchen patrol/police
LES	Leave and Earnings Statement
LOD	line of duty
LT, 1LT, 2LT	lieutenant, first lieutenant, second lieutenant
LTC	lieutenant colonel
MAJ	major

MASCAL	mass casualty
MEDCOM	Medical Command
MI	Military Intelligence
MOS	military occupational specialty
MP	military police
MRE	meal ready to eat
MRAP	mine resistant ambush protected (vehicle)
MSG	master sergeant
MTOE	Military Tables of Organization and Equipment
MWR	morale, welfare, and recreation
NBC	nuclear, biological, and chemical
NCO	noncommissioned officer
NTC	National Training Center
NWC	National War College
OCONUS	outside the continental United States
OCS	Officer Candidate School
ODP	Officer Development Program
OER	Officer Evaluation Report
OIC	officer in charge
OJT	on-the-job training
OPMS	Officer Personnel Management System
OPSEC	operational security
OPTEMPO	operation tempo (speed at which a mission is conducted)
PAM	pamphlets
PAO	public affairs officer
PAX	passengers
PBIED	person-borne improvised explosive device
PCS	permanent change of station
PERSCOM	US Total Army Personnel Command
PFC	private first class
PM	preventive maintenance
POV	privately owned vehicle
PPE	personal protective equipment
PV1	private first class
PVT	private
PX	post exchange
QM	quartermaster
R&D	research and development
RDI	regimental distinctive insignia
RHIP	rank has its privileges
ROTC	Reserve Officers' Training Corps
R&R	rest and recuperation
S1	staff officer—personnel

S2	staff officer—intelligence
S3	staff officer—training and operations
S4	staff officer—supply and logistics
SF	Special Form; Special Forces
SFC	sergeant first class
SGLI	Servicemembers Group Life Insurance
SGM	sergeant major
SGT	sergeant
SOP	standard operating procedure
SP	starting position
SPC	specialist
SPECOPS	special operations
SSG	staff sergeant
TA	Table of Allowances
TAD	temporary additional duty
TAG	the adjutant general
TD	Table of Distribution
TDA	Tables of Distribution and Allowance
TDY	temporary duty
TIG	time in grade
TIS	time in service
TLA	temporary lodging allowance
TM	Technical Manual
TOC	tactical operations center
TRADOC	US Army Training and Doctrine Command
TRANSCOM	US Transportation Command
UAV	unmanned aerial vehicle (aka drone)
UCMJ	Uniform Code of Military Justice
USA	US Army
USAF	US Air Force
USMA	United States Military Academy
USO	United Services Organization
USUHS	Uniformed Services University of the Health Sciences
UXO	unexploded ordnance
VA	US Department of Veterans Affairs
VBIED	vehicle-borne improvised explosive device (aka car bomb)
VEAP	Veterans Educational Assistance Program
VGLI	Veterans Group Life Insurance
WILCO	will comply
WO	warrant officer
WOBC	Warrant Officer Basic Course
WOCC	Warrant Office Candidate Course
XO	executive officer

Index

Page numbers in italics indicates sidebars and tables.